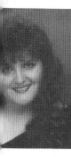

Susanne Fine, MA, RN, CS, is a Licensed Registered Nurse and a certified Psychiatric Mental-Health Clinical Nurse Specialist in private practice. She obtained two Bachelor's Degrees from Southern Oregon State College, graduating summa cum laude. She was honored at Southern Oregon State College with the ''Most Outstanding Nursing Student Award.'' Her Master's Degree in Counseling Psychology is from Lewis and Clark College and she has advanced training in Marriage/Family y. Mrs. Fine lives and works in Claremont, California where she counseling agency, ''Families In Transition.'' She also provides ing services to advanced practice nurses starting out in private .

D1291933

Springer Series on Advanced P

Terry T. Fulmer, PhD, C, FAAN,
New York University School of I

Advisory Board: Joyce Anastasi, RN, PhD; Susan
Tish Knobf, MSN, RN, FAAN; Mairead

Thera
owns
consu
practi

DEVELOPING A PRIVATE PRACTICE IN PSYCHIATRIC MENTAL-HEALTH NURSING

Susanne Fine

SPRINGER PUBLISHING COMPANY

Springer Publishing Company, Inc.
536 Broadway
New York, NY 10012-3955

Cover design by Tom Yabut and Margaret Dunin
Production Editor: Pam Ritzer

97 98 99 00 01 / 5 4 3 2 1

Library of Congress Cataloging-in-Publication Data

Fine, Susanne.
    Developing a private practice in psychiatric mental-health nursing / Susanne Fine.
        p.   cm. — (The Springer series on advanced practice nursing)
    Includes bibliographical references and index.
    ISBN 0-8261-9440-0
    1. Psychiatric nursing—Practice—United States. 2. Nurse practitioners—United States. 3. Psychotherapy—Practice—United States. I. Title.
II. Series.
    [DNLM: 1. Nursing, Private Duty. 2. Psychiatric Nursing.
3. Private Practice. WY 127 F495d 1997]
RC440.F43   1997
610.73'068—dc20
DNLM/DLC
for Library of Congress   96-33639
                                                  CIP

Printed in the United States of America

This book is dedicated to all of those nurses who have been pioneers in advanced practice.

I would also would like to express my gratitude to God who made all of this possible — for His blessings and inspiration.

May all of you support one another on your professional and personal journeys!

SUSANNE FINE M.A., R.N. , C.S.
NOVEMBER 1, 1996
CLAREMONT, CALIFORNIA

CONTENTS

PREFACE

This manual is written with the hope of sharing some of the important information that I have learned about private practice. I have been a successful nurse-therapist in private practice for seven years and have done so in Oregon, Tennessee, and California. Currently, I am a certified Clinical Nurse Specialist (American Nurses Credentialing Center/ANCC) in private practice in Claremont, California, which is about 35 miles east of Los Angeles.

I have maintained a full-time practice in California since 1991. My practice is steady, continues to grow, and I usually have a caseload of 25–30 clients. Currently, I employ three Marriage, Family, and Child Therapists, and one Psychologist. I also sublet office space to a Licensed Clinical Social Worker.

It is my hope that the advanced practice of nursing will also grow, especially the field of Psychiatric Mental-Health Nursing. I have been in nursing since 1978, and I believe that it is those of us on the front lines who will ultimately promote our profession.

It seems that there is a dearth of information about counseling practices in general, and about advanced practice nurses in private practice specifically. My intent, therefore, is to share what I know so that you, too, may contribute to the advanced practice of nursing. Furthermore, even though this book is written for nurses, it may be used by other mental-health practitioners as well. Many of the same reimbursement and practice issues are relevant. (For specific information, please contact your local licensing board and your regional professional organization.)

Throughout this book, I will stress the importance of *ethical* and *legal* practice! It is essential that you are familiar with *your* state laws and the scope of practice established by your State Board of Registered Nursing (BRN). I have included state-by-state information from each BRN, most of which will pertain, but you are ultimately responsible for keeping abreast of current changes in nursing practice. Please contact resources such as the State Board of Registered Nursing for specific questions and situations that may apply to you.

For a listing of State Boards of Nursing (SBRN) and Nurses' Associations, please see Appendix C. Always have a copy of your state laws and a copy of the rules and regulations governing your profession.

Finally, remember to share what you learn with other nurse-colleagues, so that we all may benefit from one another.

BEFORE YOU BEGIN: UNDERSTANDING REQUIREMENTS FOR PRIVATE PRACTICE

GENERAL CONSIDERATIONS

Since most states do not certify Clinical Nurse Specialists, there is usually no accurate way to know how many psychiatric mental-health clinical nurse specialists (CNS/PMHN) there are, and how many of these are in private practice. A 1992 survey from the United States Department of Health and Human Services reported that nationally there were 58,000 clinical nurse specialists (all specialties—87% employed in nursing).[1] Fewer than 10% of these were certified by the American Nurses Association (ANA).[2] This latter group cites a population of greater than 100,000 advanced practice nurses in the United States, but has no master list.[3] As of September 1995, the American Nurses Credentialing Center indicated a total of 6800 *certified* psychiatric mental-health clinical nurse specialists.[4] Of these, 6030 are adult clinical specialists and 770 are child and adolescent clinical specialists.[5] Because there is no specific exam for psychiatric nurse practitioners (NP), it is unknown at present what their numbers are. Many NPs in many states use this certification exam as criteria for nurse practitioner status.

Graduate schools of nursing began to prepare Psychiatric Nurses for independent practice in the 1960s.[6] For a complete listing of all Accredited Psychiatric Nurse Practitioner Programs, see Appendix D. In 1954, the

1

role of the CNS/PMHN was established at Rutgers University and the Nurse Training Act funded CNS training at the master's level in 1965.[7] The Social Policy Statement in 1980 included graduate education and two years later, the Council of CNSs was added to the ANA.[8]

Many nurse practice acts have been revised, and continue to be in order to accommodate the expanding role of advanced practice nurses. Some certify some or all of the four types of advanced practice nurses—nurse practitioners, nurse midwives, nurse anesthetists, and clinical nurse specialists—but it remains inconsistent. The American Nurses Association promotes state certification, but not separate licensure.[9] In late 1993, the National Council of State Boards of Nursing took the position that there should be a separate license beyond the basic RN license for all advanced practice nurses.[10] The National Council and the ANA together make recommendations to each State Board of Nursing on this issue. The confusion over whether or not to have a second license has hindered reimbursement. Even state certification does not necessarily ensure third-party payment. Although other master's-prepared clinicians have been obtaining direct reimbursement readily, nurses have been slow in reaching the same level of autonomy in third-party payments. (For a listing of states that cover reimbursement for nurses, see chapter 4.)

I collated some research statistics for the California Nurses Association (unpublished) in September of 1992, and it was distressing to see how many nurses not only knew very little about private practice specifics, but also had an extremely difficult time with third-party payment. The majority of the 100 respondents from this study were clamoring for information about these issues. Although roughly 60% were in private practices, only 60% of these received any third-party payments. Almost one-third of the group either left private practice or never went into one because of the difficulty in reimbursement. In addition, 6% said that they pursued a marriage, family, and child counselor license because of the payment difficulties. Another 19% said they billed under someone else's license.

It is hoped that some of these nurses will have access to the important information that affects practice; that is one reason why this book was written. As we expand our scope of practice, we should share what we learn, and get involved with state legislation to improve and facilitate our right to practice and receive direct reimbursement.

SOURCES OF LAW

There are four categories of law that affect the practice for psychiatric mental-health nursing. They are Constitutional Law, Statutory Provisions, Judicial Opinions, and Executive Branch Actions.[11]

Constitutional Law has to do with the Fourteenth Amendment, which states that no person shall be deprived of life, liberty, or property without due process of law. These affect commitment laws and also our right to make a fair living and not be restricted in practicing our trade.

Statutory Provisions have to do with the State's Nurse Practice Acts. These describe the authority of the nurse to practice, the scope of that practice, commitment issues, and also mandatory reporting law, such as child abuse.

Judicial Opinions interpret the status and the precepts of common law. Judges interpret the meaning of Nurse Practice Acts and others, as well as the meaning of the Fourteenth Amendment and the Bill of Rights. Negligence is also determined by courts.

Executive Branch Actions are those that are carried out to uphold the legislation. State Boards of Nursing and other licensing boards are examples of the Executive Branch. They make up the rules and regulations affecting nursing.

SCOPE OF NURSING PRACTICE

Again, it cannot be stressed enough to know the specifics of your own state nurse practice act and to have a copy of the rules and regulations. Don't hesitate to talk with your Board of Registered Nursing as well; they usually have nurse consultants there to answer your specific questions.

It is also very important that you read all of the publications put out by the American Nurses Association that directly affect your practice. One of these is the *Statement on Psychiatric and Mental Health Nurses Practice*.[12] (An extensive guide to these and other publications is found in Appendix B.)

The *Standards of Psychiatric and Mental-Health Nursing* all relate to this type of nursing in general, and specific standards such as psychotherapeutic interventions, health teaching, therapeutic environment, and psychotherapy are related to private practice.[13]

Another important document is the *Code of Nurses*.[14] This outlines the expectations that nurses will be competent and maintain credentials to perform their nursing services, show respect for human dignity, maintain confidentiality, assume responsibility for his/her actions, promote nursing, collaborate with others in a professional manner, and contribute to research and the body of knowledge in Nursing.[15]

Our responsibility is to be accountable to ourselves, our profession, and the public. In order to have high ethical standards and to maintain legality in your nursing practice, you must be informed and work with the highest level of integrity.

This means that you have the responsibility to keep abreast of current legislation and the ongoing developments in Mental Health. It also means that you should maintain your own malpractice insurance whether you are employed or working independently (see chapter 4 for details).

One of the checkpoints for accountability, which is a requisite for certification/recertification and a part of the Nursing Standards, is to have access to ongoing supervision. It is important that you have either an informal or formal contract with a supervisor. You may participate in peer-group review or meet regularly with a colleague(s), but you do not necessarily have to have on-site supervision. You do need *access* to a physician and/or other more experienced therapists with whom you can collaborate.

Some states, however, do require physician involvement or supervision, and some states require direct on-site supervision from a medical doctor. It may be acceptable for the doctor to be available by phone. The nurse may be able to work in an independent setting as long as there are written protocols that spell out specific duties and circumstances when the physician should be contacted or when the patient should be referred elsewhere.

As you can see, physician involvement can be minimal, or in the severest case, the doctor must oversee all aspects of care. Fortunately, few states are in this last category, but this is why it is critical to know the specific rules and regulations for your state. It is always important, but not mandatory, to have access to other nurse-therapists, but a psychologist, licensed clinical social worker, or marriage and family therapist will do fine as well. Peer supervision (informal) is helpful to discuss cases and legal-ethical aspects of practice. Formal supervision can also be useful and is optional as well, except as previously mentioned under "doctor supervision."

Personally, I like to meet in a small group with other mental health professionals. We all benefit from each other's perspective and there is no cost. Formal individual supervision can be done by any type of provider at a flat fee (usually $40–$120/hour). Groups supervision usually ranges from $20–$75/hour. Some of the best supervisors are those accredited by the American Association of Marriage and Family Therapists (AAMFT). They must undergo rigorous supervision training.

Finally, pick someone you can trust ethically, you like personally, and that you respect professionally. They do not necessarily need to be of the same theoretical framework as you, but it can be helpful, especially if you are doing individual therapy. Group supervision is better when the therapists do not all share the same theoretical framework.

BARRIERS TO PRACTICE

The most salient barriers to advanced practice seem to be the lack of state BRN educational and legal standards for practice and inconsistent third-party reimbursement, part of which remains the controversy over separate license versus certification.

Certification is not a standard used by every state BRN, and nurses seem to be ambivalent themselves as to its importance. On the heels of the Clinton Administration's support of expanded nurses' roles, the American Medical Association released a report opposing autonomy for advanced practice nurses.[16] The lack of sufficient knowledge of our specialty and the right to practice continues to confuse other mental and medical health providers. It also reinforces a competitive attitude toward us. This confusion also permeates our own profession and makes it easier for insurance companies to deny us status as legitimate providers.

Another barrier has been the problem of defining ourselves as nurse practitioners, versus clinical nurse specialists, versus the global term, advanced practice registered nurse. These discrepancies in titles only exacerbate and cloud our role for both consumers and providers. There are still too few graduate programs that provide adequate training in advanced roles, and there is a lack of support and confidence within nursing itself that hinders our ability to practice.

We need to share a common vision, believe in ourselves, and be determined to assert our right to provide quality, comprehensive mental-health services. Gaining support from the other three types of advanced practice nurses (nurse anesthetists, nurse midwives, and nurse practitioners) is also of paramount importance. Finally, we must join forces to enter the legal system to carve out a niche for ourselves in the legislation. Nurses generally have been shy about becoming politically active, but it is essential if we are to remain on the forefront of advanced practice. We must be willing to support our profession and to zealously safeguard the advances already won.

HOSPITAL ADMITTING PRIVILEGES

Some BRNs specifically discuss the issue of admitting privileges, but most are silent about it. Sometimes nurse-midwives and NPs are granted privileges, but not CNSs. In California, many PMHNs have admitting privileges at hospitals, but each hospital has its own by-laws that govern this process. Some hospitals are glad to give advanced practice nurses admitting privileges because of the decrease in admissions in general, and they don't want to turn down any new business. You should contact your hospital's administration to ask for admitting privileges unless your BRN says that this is prohibitive. Please note—admitting privileges are necessary in order to become part of managed care panels. Denial of privileges may be remedied by legal action, but this is costly and uncertain in outcome.[17]

CERTIFICATION

Given the hazy legal and regulatory environment, nurses should make use of the credentials nursing does offer, namely becoming certified as a clinical nurse specialist (CNS) by the American Nurses Credentialing Center (ANCC), which is a subsidiary of the American Nurses Association. The ANCC grew out of the need to organize and handle the thousands of exams taken every year. It seems to be the trend that nurses will need to be certified to be recognized as advance practice nurses. More and more states are using it as a credential for recognition of advanced practice, and it is possible that it may find its way into some state laws or scope of nursing practices. CHAMPUS (Civilian Health and Medical Program of the Uniformed Services) and other federally funded programs are using it for definition of a CNS.

As it stands now, the California BRN says that we may call ourselves certified CNSs, but they do not mandate it or say that they certify us within the state. They may eventually follow other states to include it as part of the qualifications of advanced practice. It is important to realize that if you have a master's degree outside of nursing, you no longer qualify to sit for the exam. Starting in 1994, nurses may only sit for the exam if they have a master's degree in nursing.

Furthermore, the criteria for qualified supervisors has changed. The trend will be to receive at least 65% of the supervision from nurses, so you may also charge for supervision to other nurses. This opens a new avenue of work for experienced Psychiatric Mental Health Nurses. The following are guidelines for certification of a clinical nurse specialist in adult or child psychiatric mental-health nursing.[18] You should contact the ANCC for a free certification catalog: (1-800-284-CERT). New ones are available in January of each year. The 1996 issue is no longer available; the 1997 one will be out in January.

1. Have an active RN license.
2. Be involved in direct PMHN practice an average of 4 hr/week.
3. Have access to clinical supervision/consultation.
4. Have experience in two different treatment modalities (i.e., individual, couple, or family therapy) after having completed the educational requirements below **AND**
5. a) Hold a master's degree or higher in nursing with a university identified major in psychiatric mental health nursing. A university identified major is one that is listed in the university course catalog and contains specific psychiatric and mental health nursing didactic and psychiatric and mental health nursing clinical experiences — **or — meet all of the requirements in 5b.**
    b) Hold a master's or higher degree in nursing; **AND** a minimum of 24 of graduate or post-graduate level academic credits in psychiatric and mental health theory. A minimum of 12 of these 24 graduate or post-graduate credits must contain didactic and clinical experience specific to psychiatric and mental health nursing theory. (Core courses in nursing theory, nursing research, and thesis hours will not be accepted as part of the 12 credit requirement).

    A maximum of 12 of the 24 graduate or post-graduate level credits may be in courses containing didactic and clinical experiences specific to psychiatric and mental health theory. (Examples are courses in counseling and psychology) **AND**
6. Supervised clinical training at the graduate or post-graduate level in two different treatment modalities[19] **AND**
7. Have practiced as a PMHN as follows:
    a) Have at least 800 hours of direct client contact in advanced clinical practice (up to 400 of these may have been obtained while in a master's degree clinical practicum); the other 400 must have been obtained after meeting the educational criteria in 5a or 5b.
8. Document 100 hours of individual or group clinical consultation/supervision and submit endorsement(s) from the consultant/supervisor(s) using Form A. Up to 50% of these hours must be earned following the completion of the educational preparation listed in 5a or 5b.
    a) Up to 50% of the 100 hours may be earned within a master's degree program.

b) A minimum of 65% (up to 100%) of the consultation/supervision must be provided by a nurse who is ANCC certified or is eligible for ANCC certification as a clinical specialist in psychiatric and mental health nursing. Creative alternatives are encouraged.

c) Up to 35% of the consultation/supervision may be provided by a non-nurse who meets one of the criteria listed below. (For those nurses who expect to hold prescriptive privileges, these hours might be applied toward supervision of the prescription of medications). The non-nurse(s) may be: a master's prepared licensed/certified Clinical Social Worker; A Psychiatrist; Psychologists who trained at doctoral American Psychological Association accredited programs in clinical, school, or counseling psychology; doctorally trained Psychologists who are listed in the National Registry of Health Science Providers in Psychology.

Again, please consult the catalog for detailed explanations of the above. It is a difficult exam, very complex, in a multiple-choice format. It usually takes 2–3 hours to complete. The pass rate varies, but can be as low as 62%. There are ads for study guides in the back of the *American Nurse*. I ordered two, but found them almost worthless because they were too basic, covering mostly what would be for a psychiatric nurse at a bachelor's degree level, or one working in a psychiatric hospital as a staff nurse. They were not geared toward advanced practice issues, either the legal-ethical issues or psychotherapeutic issues. The best help is the brochure from the ANCC that tells you the percentages and topics covered.

The majority of the test is supposed to cover psychotherapy, but much of it focuses on management decisions and the role of the consultation/liaison nurse. Be sure to study your mental health theories and types of therapies.

Although every exam is different, mine, which was taken in 1992, had very little pharmacology. It was very basic and was geared toward common drugs used in psychiatric hospitalizations. Most basic nursing education would meet this requirement. Because so many states do not support prescriptive privileges, the exams do not require this advanced level of psychopharmacology. This may change someday, but at present, those states that do allow for prescriptive authority require specific education and or testing at the state level, and do not involve the American Nurses Credentialing Center.

Literally, my whole test seemed to be about decision making and in order to choose the right answer, I had to know the many relevant theories. There was almost nothing on nursing diagnosis, but a fair amount was pulled from the pamphlets printed by the ANA, so I encourage you to order and read them (see Appendix B: Resources). Other practitioners who have taken the exam since 1992 have said that their exam was similar to the one that I took. Remember, you *can* take the test over again if you need to.

RECERTIFICATION

Once you have passed the exam (held twice a year in June and October), you will be notified of the results in about 6 to 8 weeks, and if you passed you will receive a certificate in 8 to 10 weeks. You will also receive a wallet card and be issued a certification number which is useful to list on your billing forms. Your certification will be good for five years. In order for you to be recertified, there are some criteria that first need to be met.

You will receive a recertification catalog about one year before your certification expires. If you meet the following recertification criteria, you do not need to sit for the exam again.

1. Have a current license as an RN; and
2. had a minimum of 1,000 hours of direct PMHN client contact during the five years since the date of certification (average 4 hours/week); and
3. had ongoing consultation/supervision since the date of certification; and
4. completed an official recertification application by:
   a) sitting for and passing the written certification exam, or
   b) presenting evidence of contact hours of continuing education or academic credit in the five years since certification (75 contact hours = 7.5 Continuing Education Unit's [CEUs], or 5 semester academic credits or 6 academic quarter credits, attendance at professional meetings, or lecturer or publication experience).

It is advantageous to obtain your recertification through continuing education so that you don't have to sit for the exam again. Most states have some form of continuing education requirement for license renewal, so you should easily be able to meet it this way. Eventually, all states may require continuing education, not just practice requirements, for licensing. It's another way to keep professional accountability. There are always changes in nursing practice, and we need to keep abreast of them. For a detailed explanation of requirements and the recertification process, please contact the ANCC (1-800-274-4ANA) for a free catalog.

SUPERVISION

Supervision or peer review is required for the certification exam, for recertification, and it is also part of our psychiatric mental-health nursing standards. Many nurses wonder what this means specifically.

First of all, you need to check with your own Board of Registered Nursing for guidelines. In California, there is no mandate that nurses have any direct supervision in order to practice, but it is part of being an accountable clinician to have ongoing consultation/peer review of your work. This does not mean that you need on-site supervision, although this may be the best for you. In private practice settings however, this may be difficult. As stated earlier, what I have done for many years is to pay for supervision in group settings and as an individual. Costs vary from $25.00 to $75.00/hr, and it can be very expensive. Since it's hard to learn new skills from someone who has less experience or training than you, some suggestions for finding supervisors are to look in your state directory of Clinical Nurse Specialists, the American Psychologists' Registry Directory, the American Association for Marriage and Family Therapists' Directory, or a local American Medical Association Psychiatry Registry. Asking other nurse therapists or clinicians who they recommend can be helpful, or you can contact your local graduate schools. As already mentioned, AAMFT supervisors are usually good. You should interview all supervisors beforehand.

It is preferable to use one supervisor if possible, even if you are in the group setting. Otherwise, you will have to have each member sign an endorsement form. (Forms and application materials are always included in the certification catalog. Remember, they are free to you.) Since it is an individual decision, many nurses will not charge for these supervision hours, but some may. However, we should try to help new graduates and others to obtain the supervision hours so that they can sit for the exam. You can still have supervision after certification from any mental-health clinician.

Always keep track of your hours of supervision; you can use the log included in this book (see chapter 3 for forms), or create your own.

Remember that supervision or consultation expenses can be tax deductible; so keep track of this as well. Having supervision once a week is ideal, but twice a month meetings work well too. Remember that if you form an association or peer support group you can count these hours as supervision, but at least one person must be a certified CNS or a licensed mental-health provider as outlined in the ANCC criteria. Another point to remember is that if you are trying to get your supervision hours (100) in order to sit for your exam, they must all be accrued before you send in your application.

AMERICAN NURSES ASSOCIATION RECOMMENDATIONS

In an article in *The American Nurse*, the American Nurses Association made the following recommendations in regard to advanced practice nursing.[20]

1. Define the nurse in advanced specialty practice.
2. Acknowledge by statute the definition of advanced specialty nursing practice and recognize professional standards and certification.
3. Recognize that regulatory systems vary and recommend:
   a) acknowledgement of advanced practice;
   b) a general definition of advanced specialty;
   c) a definition of the scope of nursing that makes reference to advanced practice to include:
      i. definitions of advanced nursing practice to include diagnosing and prescribing privileges;
      ii. provision for recognition of titles and standards;
      iii. certifying bodies guidelines;
      iv. structures and processes for reviewing and certifying certification bodies;
      v. provision for disciplinary actions.
4. Encourage state nurses associations and Boards of Nursing to jointly develop and pursue strategies to achieve the above objectives.
5. Encourage state nurses associations to promote educational opportunities for nurses in advanced practice.

6. Ensure that the ANA and SNAs continue to lobby for nondiscriminatory reimbursement for advanced practice nurses.

7. Support the development and dissemination of legislative language and administrative rules.

8. Urge the American Association of Nurse Anesthetists and the American College of Nurse Midwives to support these proposals.

This is only a brief overview, and it is helpful to understand the position of the American Nurses Association. They have great power to influence each state board of nursing and legislation, which will ultimately affect each practicing Psychiatric Mental Health Nurse.

COPING WITH A CHALLENGE TO YOUR RIGHT TO PRACTICE

It has been my personal experience that you can't be too careful. Even if you do everything with care and integrity, you may still be questioned. I had a Marriage, Family, and Child Counselor (MFCC) Intern report me to the Board of Behavioral Science Examiners (her licensing Board) for allegedly holding myself out as a MFCC. I have never used the term or the credentials; I always have worked and advertised myself as a nurse. She thought that because I did not have an MFCC license that I was misrepresenting myself and working fraudulently as an MFCC. Yet, she was incensed that nurses could do this kind of work independently without having to go through the written and oral MFCC exam. Her association also told her that nurses could not work independently without an MFCC license. (For an interesting "Letter to the Editor" about "nurses who hang out a shingle/unlicensed practice," see the *California Therapist*.[21])

My local nurse support group wrote to the editor of CAMFT with a rebuttal of "our right to practice," but there was never a redress. California seems to be particularly competitive among mental health therapists— there are over 6,000 MFCCs. The market is saturated in this state, but other states seem not to be threatened by nurse-therapists as much. The bottom line is the Board of Registered Nursing's definition and approval of the advanced practice. If you live in one of these states, then you have a stronger base for your practice and other practitioners may be more aware of the nurse's role as a therapist. Regardless, there needs to be more education within our field and with the public at large.

Because of the lack of education, I was investigated by the Board of Behavioral Science Examiners. They made a complaint to the Board of Registered Nursing, who then had to investigate me as well. Unfortunately, I was assigned an investigator from the Department of Consumer Affairs who investigated me on behalf of both Boards and who knew little about advanced practice nursing. She also questioned the BRN's authority to interpret nursing's scope of practice and seemed biased toward the Board of Behavioral Science Examiners (BBSE is the Board for MFCCs). The Rules and Regulations handbook for the BBSE states in section 4980.01, pp. 2–3, "nothing in this chapter shall be construed to constrict, limit, or withdraw the . . . Nurse Practice Act."[22] The other professional Practice Acts are included here. Otherwise, every other mental health professional would need a MFCC license as well as their own license for their profession. The BRN has been strong in backing me and other advanced practice nurses in maintaining our right to practice.

Since I have been in accordance with the law and within my scope of nursing practice, I will not be prosecuted for counseling without an MFCC license because we as nurses may legally perform these services under our nursing license. The Board of Registered Nursing puts out a position paper that addresses the scope of psychiatric mental-health nursing in California. (You can contact them for a copy.) This issue has been going on for years. As more nurses move out into areas of practice that are new and that overlap other professions, besides medicine, we will continue to be challenged. This is one of the reasons that this book was written—to help you be aware of these issues, and to help you to be well informed and accountable. Please see "Strategies for Right to Practice," in *The Nurse Psychotherapist in Private Practice*,[23] for important legal cases. The California Nurses Association is also strongly aware and supportive of advanced practice as it relates to psychiatric mental-health nursing.

As it stands now, the California Attorney General is looking at this issue. Part of the dilemma involves the fact that the California BRN has a broad scope of nursing practice that has been written to accommodate changes within the field and that has permeable boundaries.[24] It has been written very broadly to adjust to the changes in the practice that make it difficult for nonnurses to assess whether or not a function is within the scope of nursing practice.

The California BRN has said that we can use the term counselor or counseling, psychiatric mental-health nurse, and we may say we are certified by ANA if applicable. I did not find this type of limitation when practicing in Oregon or Tennessee. Furthermore, it is prudent that the CBRN says that we cannot perform services for which we are not fully trained, even if they are within our scope of practice. A copy of the

Insurance Codes (Table 1.1) follows the national summary (see pp. 20–24). The best way to prevent challenges to your right to practice is to be well informed of your state's requirements for practice and the practice acts. The following section and Appendix A provide an overview of this information. If you are contacted by any licensing board, even the Board of Registered Nursing, then the following guidelines may be helpful.

1) Contact the BRN and speak to a nurse-consultant about the rules and regulations regarding specific rights to practice. Have them sent to you in writing if possible.

2) Call the Enforcement Division within the BRN and speak to someone who is handling your case. Ask specifically what their concerns are and why the investigation is being done, such as, patient/consumer complaint, other regulatory Board complaint, or other health practitioner complaint.

3) Call the State Nurses Association to ask for a lawyer referral (try to find one who is a nurse). It is not necessary to be a member to do this. You can also call The American Nurses Association and talk to their legal department as well. David Keepnews RN, JD is in charge there. Both of these organizations are eager to hear of any advanced practice nurses being harassed.

4) Be sure to find a lawyer who works with the Department of Consumer Affairs (agency that handles complaints from the consumers involving medical professionals) to inform you of your rights. It may be titled something different in your state, but the BRN will have this information. Try to get as many facts about your case as possible, including any written complaints, copies of your file, etc.

5) If scheduled for a hearing with the Department of Consumer Affairs, be sure to bring legal representation even if they tell you it is not needed. Do not agree to tape recording the meeting/investigation if possible. Be prepared that the investigator may not be educated about advanced practice; they usually have a police, not nursing, background.

The meeting/investigation will determine if there is a case against you. If so, the case will be filed against you with the District Attorney. It will not automatically go to court because the DA's office must find just cause that the laws are being broken. In my case, the Department of Consumer Affairs (from the BBSE side, not the BRN's) wanted to pursue prosecution, but the district attorney investigator could find no case.

Try really hard to get things in writing; it may be very difficult even if they drop the case. Most BRNs do not keep anything in your file unless some negative disposition occurs, such as court proceedings, so that if someone calls and checks on your license it will be free from complaints or charges.

NATIONAL SUMMARY OF LEGAL REQUIREMENTS FOR PRACTICE FOR ADVANCED PRACTICE NURSES

This section will summarize practice and educational requirements for APNs in the United States. For more detailed descriptions of the requirements of individual states, see Appendix A.

Recognition of Advanced Practice

All states legislatively recognize advanced practice except for Illinois, Minnesota, Pennsylvania, and Tennessee. Despite this, APNs may practice anyway in these states under expanded roles from a broad Nurse Practice Act.

Independent Practice

APNs may work completely independently of physicians in in the following states:

Alaska	Indiana	Oregon
Arizona	Maine	Rhode Island
Colorado	Maryland	South Carolina
Connecticut	Michigan	Texas
Delaware	Montana	Utah
District of Columbia	New Hampshire	Vermont
Hawaii	New Mexico	Virginia
Kansas	North Dakota	Washington
Iowa	Oklahoma	West Virginia

Scope of Practice

There are 20 states where APNs have complete autonomy over their practice. This includes: independent practice setting, BRN statutes that recognize APNs (including CNSs), prescriptive privileges, and the ability to be reimbursed by third-party payors (including legislation). They are:

Alaska	Massachusetts*	Rhode Island*
Arizona	Montana	South Carolina*
Colorado	New Hampshire	Texas*
Connecticut*	New Mexico	Utah*
Delaware	North Dakota	Vermont*
District of Columbia	Oklahoma	West Virginia*
Iowa	Oregon	

*These states have minimal physician involvement with prescriptive privileges, i.e., protocols, collaboration, or written guidelines. Despite this, APNs may still practice in independent settings.

CNSs

Most states legislatively recognize NPs, CRNSs, CNMs, and CNSs. The states that do not define or recognize CNSs are: California, Idaho, Illinois, Michigan, Mississippi, Nebraska, New York, North Carolina, Oregon, Pennsylvania, and Tennessee. CNSs may practice despite this in California, Michigan, Oregon, and Tennessee. Some states recognize only psychiatric CNSs. They are: Florida, Georgia, Maryland, Massachusetts, Minnesota, Nevada, New Hampshire, Vermont, and Washington.[25] California calls them PMHNs.

Prescriptive Privileges

All states allow for prescriptive privileges for APNs (not necessarily all types) except for Illinois and Ohio. Some states do mandate that APNs have physician supervision or collaboration when utilizing prescriptive privileges, even if their practice is autonomous otherwise. Please contact your BRN for specific prescriptive privilege guidelines. Ohio allows for prescriptive privileges under physician supervision, protocols, and only in specified university pilot projects.

The following four states also mandate malpractice insurance for the APN who elects to practice with prescriptive privileges:[26,27] Florida, Mississippi, Wisconsin, and Wyoming. DEA numbers are available in 24 states:[28]

Alaska	Montana	Pennsylvania
Arizona	Nebraska	Rhode Island
Connecticut	Nevada	South Carolina
District of Columbia	New Hampshire	Utah

Iowa	New Mexico	Vermont
Maine	New York	Washington
Maryland	North Carolina	West Virginia
Massachusetts	North Dakota	Wisconsin
Minnesota	Oregon	Wyoming

Prescriptive privileges allow for nurses to write a prescription for noncontrolled and controlled drugs depending on regulations. Controlled substances under the DEA include Schedule (II–V), the lower number having the greatest risk of abuse/dependence.[29,30] Noncontrolled or legend drugs are other medicines, i.e., antibiotics, cardiac medication, insulin, etc. The following fifteen states allow for prescriptive authority to APNs, excluding controlled substances: Alabama, California (LP), Florida (LP), Idaho (LP), Hawaii, Kansas, Kentucky (LP), Louisiana, Michigan, Mississippi, Missouri, Nevada, New Jersey, Tennessee, and Texas.

Thirty-eight states allow prescriptive privileges for CNSs:

Alaska	Kentucky	Oklahoma
Arizona	Louisiana	Pennsylvania (LP)
Arkansas	Maine	South Carolina
Colorado	Massachusetts	Tennessee
Connecticut	Michigan	Texas
Delaware	Minnesota	Utah
District of Columbia	Missouri	Vermont
Florida	Montana	Virginia
Hawaii	Nevada	Washington
Indiana	New Hampshire	Wisconsin
Iowa	New Jersey	West Virginia
Georgia	New Mexico	Wyoming
Kansas	North Dakota	

The following states allow for prescriptive privileges for APNs, excluding CNSs: Alaska, California, Idaho, Maryland, Mississippi, Nebraska, New York, North Carolina, Oregon, Rhode Island, and South Dakota.

Third-Party Reimbursement

Twenty-one states do not have legislative mandates for third-party reimbursement, excluding MediCaid and/or MediCare reimbursement. They are: Alabama, Arkansas, District of Columbia, Georgia, Hawaii, Idaho, Illinois, Kansas, Kentucky, Louisiana, Missouri, Nebraska, New York,

Ohio, Oklahoma, Pennsylvania, South Carolina, Texas, Vermont, Utah, and Wisconsin (LP). Each state summary delineates MediCaid and/or MediCare coverage.

Reimbursement Legislation

There are 30 states that have specific legislation in place or pending that assists with third-party reimbursement for APNs. Not all types of APNs are listed in each of these insurance laws. And even though the mandates exist, there is almost universal difficulty for APNs to become part of managed care panels (PPOs, EAPs, and HMOs). Also, these mandates do not always ensure reimbursement from the other types of payors (private indemnity, self-insured, Blue Cross/Blue Shield, MediCaid, and MediCare). Most BRNs do not have much information regarding this. The following nine states are reporting that APNs are being reimbursed and included in managed care systems: Arizona, California, Florida, Kansas (LP), Kentucky, Maryland, Mississippi, New Hampshire, and North Dakota (LP). The main barrier to APN reimbursement from managed care companies is that laws are written too narrowly, and most managed care companies do not have to follow the state's insurance codes. Instead, they fall under the jurisdiction of the Department of Corporations. Many states have anti-discrimination and anti-trade language in their Insurance laws and Health & Safety Codes, yet managed care seems to be without accountability in this area. For a thoughtful article on APNs and managed care, please see Marcia Lepler's, ''Managed care brings APNs mixed blessings.[31,32]

APNs must join together to ensure a place in managed care or they will find that all of the successes in advancing nursing will be overshadowed by the lack of availability to patients and communities because APNs cannot be reimbursed for their services.

Despite the managed care issues, there are 30 states that have specific legislation in place or pending that assist with third-party reimbursement for APNs. Not all types of APNs are listed in each of these insurance laws. Almost nothing is written into these laws mandating managed care to be included. Some only have legislative assistance for MediCaid and/ or MediCare. The states are:

Alaska	Massachusetts	North Dakota
Arizona	Michigan	Oregon
California	Minnesota	Pennsylvania
Colorado	Mississippi	Rhode Island

Connecticut	Montana	Tennessee (LP)
Delaware	Nevada	Virginia
Florida	New Hampshire	Washington
Iowa (LP)	New Jersey	West Virginia
Maine	New Mexico	Wisconsin (LP)
Maryland	North Carolina	Wyoming

All in all, the last 2–3 years have brought enormous advances in legislation and BRN guidelines for APNs.[33] Each January, *The Nurse Practitioner: The American Journal of Primary Health Care* prints national updates on legislative, reimbursement, and prescriptive privileges changes. Although most state Nurse Practice Acts have included NPs, CNMs, and RNAs for some time, CNSs are just now being added. The major reason behind this is that they have been primarily in acute care settings, but now are moving into more out-patient and private practice settings. This will certainly open up many opportunities for CNSs who are the largest growing type of APN. Specifically, the psychiatric CNS is the subspecialty that has the biggest CNS population and is expanding the fastest.

The biggest barrier still seems to be the reimbursement issue. It seems essential that each state provide for specific legislation which mandates third-party reimbursement for all of the types of APNs. Without this, APNs are being reimbursed inconsistently. Without third-party payment, many APNs will not be able to survive economically, especially in this age of competitive managed care. It also seems to follow that if a provider receives third-party reimbursement, then he/she is more likely to be accepted by the public and professional community. Nurses have been shy about pushing for their right for reimbursement and also about being involved in the legislative area. These two areas are essential for the survival of advanced practice. I encourage all of you to work with your state BRN and Nurses Association to alleviate barriers to practice. Again, it is hoped that some national guidelines will be developed so that each state will have comparable standards so that APNs may move about freely from state to state without hampering their ability to practice. If we as a profession can standardize our practice in terms of titles, education, certification, and practice requirements, then we can begin to educate the public and other health professions about advanced practice. Because each new year brings legislative changes, please keep current by being in touch with your state Nurses Association and BRN for changes.

TABLE 1.1   California Insurance Code

Division 2. Classes of Insurance
Part 2. Life and Disability Insurance
Chapter 1. The Contract
Article 4. Payment and Proceeds

10176. Medical Reimbursement Provisions of Disability Policies; Selection of Certificate Holder or Licensee; Unenforceability of Waiver of Mental Health Services Coverage.

In disability insurance, the policy may provide for payment of medical, surgical, chiropractic, physical therapy, speech pathology, audiology, acupuncture, professional mental health, dental, hospital, or optometric expenses upon a reimbursement basis, or for the exclusion of any such services, and provision may be made therein for payment of all or a portion of the amount of charge for these services without requiring that the insured first pay the expenses. No such policy shall prohibit the insured from selecting any psychologist, or other person who is the older of a certificate or license under Section 1000, 1634, 2135, 2553, 2630, 2948, 3055 or 4938 of the business and Professions Code to perform the particular services covered under the terms of the policy, the certificate holder or licensee being expressly authorized by law to perform such services.

If the insured selects any person who is a holder of a certificate under Section 4938 of the business and Professions Code, a disability insurer or nonprofit hospital service plan shall pay the bona fide claim of an acupuncturist holding a certificate pursuant to Section 4938 of the business and Professions Code for the treatment of an insured person only if the insured's policy or contract expressly includes acupuncture as a benefit and includes coverage for the injury or illness treated. Unless the policy or contract expressly includes acupuncture as a benefit, no person who is the holder of any license or certificate set forth in this section shall be paid or reimbursed under such policy for acupuncture.

Nor shall any such policy prohibit the insured, upon referral by a physician and surgeon licensed under Section 2135 of the Business and Professions Code from selecting any licensed clinical social worker who is the holder of a license issued under Section 9040 of the Business and Professions Code; or any occupational therapist as specified in Section 2570 of the Business and Professions Code; or any marriage, family, and child counselor who is the holder of a license under section 4980.50 of the Business and Professions Code, to perform the particular services covered under the terms of the policy; or from selecting any speech pathologist or audiologist licensed under Section 2530 of the Business and Professions Code or any registered nurse licensed pursuant to Chapter 6 (commencing with Section 2700) of Division 2 of the Business and Professions Code who possesses a master's degree in psychiatric mental-health nursing, at such time as the State Board of Registered Nurses produces and maintains a list of those psychiatric mental-health nurses who possess a master's degree in psychiatric mental-health nursing, to perform services deemed necessary by the referring physicians, such certificate holder, licensee or otherwise regulated person, being expressly authorized by law to perform the services.

Nothing in this section shall be construed to allow any certificate holder or licensee enumerated in this section to perform professional mental health services beyond his or her field or fields of competence as established by his or her education, training, and experience. For the purposes of this section, ''marriage, family, and child counselor'' means a licensed marriage, family, and child counselor who has received specific instruction in assessment, diagnosis, prognosis, and counseling, and psychotherapeutic treatment of premarital, marriage, family, and child relationship dysfunctions which is equivalent to the instruction required for licensure on January 1, 1981. 10176.7 Disability insurance written or issued for delivery outside state; selection of California licensed clinical social worker, registered psychiatric mental health nurse or marriage, family and child counselor.

Disability insurance where the insurer is licensed to do business in this state and which provides coverage under a contract of insurance which includes California residents but which may be written or issued for delivery outside of California where benefits are provided within the scope of practice of a licensed clinical social worker, a registered nurse licensed pursuant to Chapter 6 (commencing with Section 2700) of Division 2 of the Business and Professions Code who possesses a master's degree in psychiatric mental-health nursing and two years of supervised experience in psychiatric mental-health nursing, or a marriage, family, and child counselor who is the holder of a license under Section 17805 of the Business and professions Code, shall not be deemed to prohibit persons covered under the contract from selecting those licensees in California to perform the services in California which are within the terms of the contract even through the licensees are not licensed in the state where the contract is written or issued for delivery.

It is the intent of the Legislature in amending this section in the 1984 portion of the 1983–1984 Legislative Session that persons covered by the insurance and those providers of health care specified in this section who are licensed in California should be entitled to the benefits provided by the insurance for services of those providers rendered to those persons.

10177. Mental health coverage in self-insured employee welfare benefit plan; unenforceability of waiver of lifetime coverage.

A self-insured employee welfare benefit plan may provide for payment of professional mental health expenses upon a reimbursement basis, or for the exclusion of such services and provision may be made therein for payment of all or a portion of the amount of charge for such services without requiring that the employee first pay such expenses. No such plan shall prohibit the employee from selecting any psychologist who is the holder of a certificate issued under Section 2948 of the Business and Professions Code or, upon referral by a physician and surgeon licensed under Section 2135 of the Business and Professions Code, any licensed clinical social worker who is the holder of a license issued under Section 9040 of the Business and Professions Code or any marriage, family, and child counselor who is the holder of a certificate of license under Section 4980.50 of the Business and Professions Code, or any registered nurse licensed pursuant to Chapter 6 (commencing with Section 2700) of division 2 of the Business and Professions Code who possesses a master's degree in psychiatric mental-health nursing and two years of supervised experience in psychiatric mental-health nursing and two years of supervised experience in psychiatric mental-health nursing, at such time as the State Board of Registered Nurses produces and maintains a list of those psychiatric mental-health nurses who possess a master's degree in psychiatric-mental health nursing and two years supervised experience in psychiatric mental-health nursing, to perform the particular services covered under the terms of the plan, such certificate or license holder being expressly authorized by law to perform such services.

(Continued)

Any individual disability insurance policy, which is issued, renewed, or amended on or after January 1, 1988, which includes mental health services coverage may not include a lifetime waiver for that coverage with respect to any applicant. The lifetime waiver of coverage provision shall be deemed unenforceable.

Nothing in this section shall be construed to allow any certificate holder or licensee enumerated in this section to perform professional services beyond his or her field or fields of competence as established by his or her education, training, and experience. For the purposes of this section, "marriage, family and child counselor" shall mean a licensed marriage, family and child counselor who has received specific instruction in assessment, diagnosis, prognosis, and counseling, and psychotherapeutic treatment of premarital, marriage, family and child relationship dysfunctions which is equivalent to the instruction required for licensure on January 1, 1981.

A self-insured employee welfare benefit plan, which is issued, renewed, or amended on or after January 1, 1988, which includes mental health services coverage in nongroup contracts may not include a lifetime waiver for that coverage with respect to any employee. the lifetime waiver of coverage provision shall be deemed unenforceable.

10177.8. Self-insured employee welfare benefit plans written or issued for delivery outside state; selection of California licensed clinical social worker, registered psychiatric mental health nurse or marriage, family and child counselor.

A self-insured employee welfare benefit plan doing business in this state and which provides coverage which includes California resident but which may be written or issued for delivery outside of California where benefits are provided within the scope of practice of a licensed clinical social worker, a registered nurse licensed pursuant to Chapter 6 (commencing with Section 2700) of Division 2 of the Business and Professions Code who possesses a master's degree in psychiatric mental-health nursing, or a marriage, family, and child counselor who is the holder of a license under Section 17805 of the Business and Professions Code, shall not be deemed to prohibit persons covered under the plan from selecting those licensees in California to perform the Services in California which are within the terms of the contact even though the licensees are not licensed in the state where the contract is written or issued.

It is the intent of the Legislature in amending this section of the 1984 portion of the 1983–1984 Legislative Session that persons covered by the plan and those providers of health care specified in this section who are licensed in California should be entitled to the benefits provided by the plan for services of those providers rendered to those persons.

CHAPTER 11a. NONPROFIT HOSPITAL SERVICE PLANS
Article 6. The Contract.

11512.3 Required Provisions of master contract.

Every group master hospital service contract issued under the terms of Section 11512.2 shall contain the following provisions.

(a) A provision that the contract, the application of the employer, or the executive officer or trustee or any association or trustees, and the individual applications, if any of the employees or members covered shall constitute the entire contract between the parties and that all statements made by the employer, or the executive officer, or trustee or trustees, or by the individual employee or members shall, in the absence of fraud, be deemed representations and not warranties, and that no such statement shall be used in defense to a claim under the contract, unless it is contained in a written application;

(b) A provision that the corporation will issue to the employer or to the executive officer or trustee of the association or to the trustees, for delivery to each of the employees or members who are covered under such contract, an individual certificate setting forth a statement as to the hospital service to which he is entitled;

(c) A provision that to the group or class thereof originally covered shall be added from time to time all new employees of the employer or members of the association eligible to and applying for coverage in such group or class;

(d) A statement that such contract is not in lieu of and does not affect any requirement or coverage by workmen's compensation insurance;

(e) Such provisions as may be promulgated by the commissioner from time to time. (Amended by Stats. 1974, Ch. 544, p. Sect. 35).

11512.8 Professional mental health coverage; unenforceability of waiver of mental health services coverage

A hospital service contract may provide for payment of professional mental health expenses upon a reimbursement basis, or for the exclusion of such services, and provision may be made therein for payment of all or a portion of the amount of charge for such services without requiring that the employee first pay such expenses. No such contract shall prohibit the subscriber from selecting any psychologist who is the holder of a certificate issued under Section 2948 of the Business and Professions Code or, upon referral by a physicians and surgeon licensed under Section 2135 of the Business and Professions Code, any licensed clinical social worker who is the holder of a license issued under Section 9040 of the Business and Professions Code or any marriage, family and child counselor who is the holder of a license under Section 4980.50 of the Business and Professions Code or any registered nurse licensed pursuant to Chapter 6 (commencing with Section 2700) of Division 2 of the Business and Professions code who possesses a master's degree in psychiatric mental-health nursing and two years of supervised experience in psychiatric mental-health nursing, to perform the particular services covered under the terms of the contract, such certificate or license holder being expressly authorized by law to perform such services.

Nothing in this section shall be construed to allow any certificate holder or licensee enumerated in this section to perform professional mental health services beyond his or her field or fields of competence as established by his or her education, training, and experience. For the purposes of this section, "marriage, family, and child counselor" shall mean a licensed marriage, family, and child counselor who has received specific instruction in assessment, diagnosis, prognosis, and counselor and psychotherapeutic treatment of premarital, marriage, family and child relationship dysfunctions which is equivalent to the instruction required for licensure on January 1, 1981.

(Continued)

TABLE 1.1 *(Continued)*
A hospital service contract, which is issued, renewed, or amended on or after January 1, 1988, which includes mental health services coverage in non-group contracts may not contain a lifetime waiver for that coverage with respect to any applicant. The lifetime waiver of coverage provision shall be deemed unenforceable.

NOTES

1. Gray, B. B. (1994, August). Clinical nurse specialists to be studied by BRN. *Nurseweek, 7*(17), 16.
2. Ibid.
3. Meehan, J. (1994, January). ANA expresses disappointment over AMA opposition to APN autonomy. *The American Nurse*, 1.
4. Hammers, M. Psych Nurses. (July 21). *RN Times*.
5. American Nurses Credentialing Center. (1996). *American Nurses Credentialing Center Certification Catalog.* Washington, DC: Author.
6. Sebastian, L. (1991). Third party reimbursement for nurses in advanced practice. *Perspectives in Psychiatric Care, 27*, 7.
7. Gray, 16.
8. California Board of Registered Nursing. (1994). *Clinical Nurse Specialist Task Force Memo.*
9. American Nurses Association, (1993). *ANA Council Perspectives, 2*, 7.
10. Ibid.
11. Durham, J., & Hardin, S. (Eds.). (1986). *The nurse psychotherapist in private practice.* New York: Springer Publishing.
12. American Nurses Association. (1994). *Statement on psychiatric and mental health nursing practice.* Kansas City: Author.
13. Ibid.
14. American Nurses Association. (1985). *Code for nurses.* Kansas City: Author.
15. Ibid.
16. Meehan, 1.
17. Moss, R. (1993, November/December). ''Privileging Essential to APN autonomy.'' *American Nurse*, 7.
18. American Nurses Credentialing Center. (1996). *ANCC Certification Catalog.* Washington, DC: Author, pgs. 20–23. Reprinted by permission.
19. ANA, ''Certification exam requirements change,'' *American Nurse,* July/August 1994, 31.
20. American Nurses Association. (1993, February). *The American Nurse*, 22.
21. California Association for Marriage and Family Therapists. (Nov/Dec, 1992). *California Therapist.*
22. State of California Department of Consumer Affairs. (1990). Laws and regulations relating to the practice of marriage, family, and child counseling. Sacramento, CA: Author.

23. Durham, J., & Hardin, S. (1986).
24. California Nurses Association. (1989). *Nursing Practice in California: Rights, Responsibilities, and Regulations* (2nd ed.). San Francisco: Author.
25. Pearson, L. (Ed.). (1996, January). Annual Update of how each state stands on legislative issues affecting advanced nursing practice. *The Nurse Practitioner,* 10–70.
26. American Psychiatric Nurses Association. (1996, July). Prescriptive authority chart. Congress on Advanced Practice in Psychiatric Nursing, 1–8.
27. Carson, W. (1996, February). Prescriptive authority chart. American Nurses Association Nurse Practice Counsel, 1–8.
28. Ibid.
29. Ibid.
30. Huff, B. (Ed.). (1996). *Physician's Desk Reference.* Oradell, NJ: Litton Industries, 2687.
31. Lepler, M. (September 2, 1996). Managed care brings APNs mixed blessings (Part 1). *NURSEweek,* 1, 22–23.
32. Lepler, M. (September 16, 1996). Managed care brings APNs mixed blessings (Part 2). *NURSEweek,* 1, 22.
33. Pearson, 10–70.

PLANNING THE SCOPE OF YOUR PRACTICE

PLANNING

First, you need to assess how important a private practice is to you. It will take hard work and determination if you want to succeed, and if your desire is not strong, you may not be able to pull it off.

Start by asking yourself what you would most like in a job. Would you deal well with autonomy, flexible work hours, and not having a regular paycheck? Do you work well alone? Is marketing a four-letter word to you? Do you have the patience to make it work? If you think that you can manage the anxiety of not knowing when your income will be steady, if you like setting your own schedule, and you enjoy being autonomous and working on your own, then a private practice may be for you.

Planning and marketing your practice is an important step to having a successful business. To ensure client referrals on an ongoing basis, you must have good referral sources that are consistent. In order to achieve this, you must do many things.

Determining Your Scope of Practice

First, you must develop a philosophy or theory that guides your practice so that when asked, "What is a nurse therapist?", or "What is it that you do?'', you can respond intelligently. Many nurses and most of the public and other medical or mental-health professionals are not aware of what a clinical nurse specialist is, or what kind of counseling services we perform. The public is much more familiar with nurse practitioners. So, it is important that you have a keen grasp on what theoretical bases your nursing practice is founded.

Theory is evolved from the Greek word *theoria*, which translates to ''vision.'' Without a vision or awareness of important theories guiding your practice, it will be hard to be accountable to yourself and the clients. Review the following nurse theories, and others, to decipher who has influenced your work the most: Hildegard Peplau—Interpersonal Model; Dorothea Orem—Self-care Model; Imogene King—Goal Attainment Model; Dorothy Johnson—Behavioral Systems Model; Martha Rogers— Unitary Person Model; and Sister Callista Roy—Adaptation Model. Others that may be useful include: Nightingale, Hall, Henderson, Abdellah, Wiedenbach, and Levine.[1] Other theories from various disciplines that your practice may use can be broken down into the following categories: Stress, Developmental, Family/Systems, Interactive, Adaptation, Role, Change, and Need. If necessary, review counseling theories from coursework that you have taken, or get a good counseling theories text from a graduate program bookstore.

After you decide which theories have influenced you the most, then you must ask yourself the following questions. It may be helpful if you write these questions—and your answers—in a journal: How do you identify problems? Why do people need therapy? How do people change? What theories do you draw from? What are the principal concepts of your theory? What role do you see yourself in? What is your process of doing therapy? How do you evaluate the effectiveness of your therapy? How are you different from other mental-health professionals? What type of clients do you want to work with? For example, children and families interest you a lot. Or, you have special experience working with women who have been sexually molested as children. What special populations or type of problems do you have unique experience or training in? It is helpful for you to work with people in which you have a natural interest. Do not work with clients that behave in ways that are intolerable or where you can't be objective or nonjudgmental, such as sexual offenders. You must understand your own limitations. Refer those clients that you cannot work with to other therapists. Give them three sources to contact if possible, especially professionals with whom you have personal knowledge.

Another aspect of this journey that would be helpful would be to meet with another nurse colleague to share your nursing theory and practice.

This will help you to answer more confidently when a client or other professional asks you what you do.

Marketing

I always start my initial session with a client by describing to them what I do and what my role is as a clinical nurse specialist. I also do this in an abbreviated form when talking to a prospective client over the phone. For example, I discuss my nursing education and medical background. A few points to help elucidate the differences of a nursing perspective are that nursing differs from other disciplines in its holistic approach to care, that is, the mind-body-spirit approach to health. Nursing uses a preventative approach, not just restorative interventions. It is also educative, teaching the client to care for self. It is also systemic and looks at treating the whole family within a broader community system. I discuss that my personal approach is directive, and that I take a very active role in my therapy. (This depends mostly on the theoretical framework that guides the individual nurse's therapy.)

Always remember: Each contact that you have with the public or another professional is an opportunity to market yourself! Furthermore, I believe it is our duty as nurses to provide information to the public about our expanding role as advanced practice nurses. We must do this thoughtfully and with great care.

It may help if you think of marketing as nothing more than educating others about who you are and what it is that you do. In reality, you are teaching and giving information. More nursing programs should help graduate nursing students to confront this issue before getting out into practice.

Self-Promotion

Many nurses are generally squeamish about this aspect of having a private practice; they feel uncomfortable about promoting their services or advertising. If you don't tell others about yourself, though, then how will they know to come to see you instead of the other mental-health professionals out there?

Why see a nurse therapist instead of a psychiatrist, psychologist, social worker, or marriage, family, and child counselor? I have developed a fact sheet on clinical nurse specialists to hand out to clients and insurance companies. (See Table 2.1.) Please be creative and make your own or adapt the one in this book to suit your personal needs.

TABLE 2.1   What is a Clinical Nurse Specialist in Psychiatric Mental-Health Nursing?

This fact sheet is designed to describe the scope of practice for those registered nurses who are adequately trained and experienced to perform therapy and counseling services under California law.

All active registered nurses are required to be licensed and to meet stringent educational and experience requirements. Registered nurses with master's degrees in psychiatric mental-health nursing or in counseling may provide therapy and counseling to individuals, couples, and families utilizing a broad range of psychotherapeutic techniques. Usually, these nurses are referred to as clinical nurse specialists or psychiatric mental health nurses. They may choose to be nationally certified as such by exam after meeting the necessary criteria in education and experience.

Clinical nurse specialists have a unique background that allows them to understand the physical, psychological, pharmacological, and social processes that affect the client and family. They draw upon information and research from a variety of fields including nursing, medicine, sociology, psychology, marriage/family therapy, and others. Nurses who have advanced training may specialize in working with children/adolescents, family therapy, substance abuse, sexual abuse, and so on. Furthermore, psychiatric mental health nurses may work independently or with other professionals in a variety of settings which include private practice, clinics, community mental-health centers, and hospitals.

In 1982, California passed legislation mandating private insurance reimbursement for mental health services by master's-prepared psychiatric mental health nurses who have two years of supervised experience. The Board of Registered Nursing has provided that these qualified registered nurses may be listed with them and be given a provider number. Many nurses do not choose to be listed with the Board of Registered Nursing, but are still legally authorized to perform counseling services and to bill insurance companies directly. An important goal for psychiatric mental health nurses is to provide quality care to clients in order to promote both physical and mental health and well-being using preventative, educative, restorative, and therapeutic techniques that follow professional, legal, and ethical guidelines. The psychiatric mental health nurse is a skilled and knowledgeable health care provider, and has the responsibility to assess and care for the total client. These advanced practitioners are required to seek out continual education, supervision, and consultation which will promote quality nursing care and accountability.

Another important key to marketing is being sure to describe how your services are cost-effective and of high quality because of the unique training and education that you have had. Be sure to point out that nursing is comprehensive in scope. With so many mental-health professionals in the field, you must assert your specialness with confidence, but first you must believe in yourself. If you lack confidence or have low self-esteem, then get help from other nurse colleagues. Look at who else is in the field. Find yourself a mentor. It also could be very helpful to join a support group or create your own. There are six that I know of in the California area:

The Association of Psychiatric Mental
Health Advanced Practice Nurses
715 W. Foothill Blvd.
Glendora, CA 91740
Contact: Grace Farnham, MSN, RN, CS
(818) 339-3727

The Association of Psychiatric Mental Health
Nurses in Private Practice,
12021 Wilshire Blvd, Suite 797
Los Angeles, CA 90025
Contact: Virginia Wittig, MSN, RN (310) 364-0960

San Diego Society of Specialists
in Psychiatric-Mental Health Nursing
4864 Bradshaw St.
San Diego, CA 92130
Contact: Margo Wilson
(619) 943-8681

Northern California Chapter
Contact: Judith Beel, MSN, RN
(415) 329-9119

Ventura County-Ojai Chapter
Contact: Barabara Antonelli, PhD., RN, CS
(805) 648-5191

Sacramento Chapter
Contact: Bonnie Walker or Arlene Bruinsma
(916) 569-8680

All of these groups meet on a monthly or bi-monthly basis. You should join or find out about a group in your own area. Don't be afraid to start your own because we all need support and the sharing of information. Networking is essential to developing our advanced practice.

Specific Strategies

After having become comfortable in presenting your ideas about your practice, and setting up your office, you can begin to develop some specific marketing strategies. First, ask yourself if there is a special population that you want to work with, such as children. Then ask yourself if there is a special type of problem that you want to work with, for example, sexual abuse. Then, find out where this population and/or problem exists the most.

Is this something that is already being treated in your local area, and by whom? Think of specific ways that you can begin to network and to let this population know that you are available. The following, although not an exhaustive one, is a listing of some ideas for contacts that may be helpful to you. You should develop an ongoing list for yourself.

Pastors/churches

Daycare, elementary, and secondary schools

College or high school counseling centers

Rotary club, Lions club, etc.

Other nurses or medical/mental-health professionals

Battered womens' shelters

Sexual assault centers

Help-Line community counseling referrals

Alcoholics Anonymous and other 12-step groups

Parents without Partners

Foster Parents or Step-Parents of America

Local hospitals or clinics

Employee assistance programs at businesses

Newspapers or local magazines

Nursing journals or newspapers

Nursing schools

YWCA or YMCA

Friends/relatives/business contacts

Workshops or seminars

Any public speaking opportunity

Professional associations

Directories of any kind

Insurance/managed care companies listing

Local managed care assessors

Radio or television advertisements/talk shows

Local ads/bulletins on display

Any volunteer organizations/self-help groups

Volunteering your time

Your own personal doctor, dentist, etc.

American Diabetes Assoc./AHA, other special groups

Local phone book/yellow page ads/listings

Teaching local classes in community/colleges

Senior Citizens Center

Local Hospitals, clinics, and nursing homes

Career Days at high schools and colleges

Client's personal minister and physicians

These are just a few suggestions and must be tailored to your personal practice specialty and interests. Always ask your client how they heard of you, and once you do get a referral, always follow it up with an immediate thank-you note to the referral source (after you have permission from the client).

Setting Up Meetings

After you have decided who your potential contacts will be, then you can start arranging to meet with them in person, and/or contact them over the phone. A good rule of thumb in marketing is to realize that a person usually will not remember you until they have either heard your name or seen it in print about five or six times. So it is important that after meeting with someone, you give them a business card or a brochure, and follow up your phone calls with something in writing (a nice cover letter along with brochure, business card, resume, etc.). (A sample brochure is shown in Figure 2.1, and a sample business card is shown in Figure 2.2.) Be sure to send a note or letter saying thanks to those who did meet with you in person or had lunch with you.

One of the best techniques seems to be calling someone and then asking to treat them to lunch where you can get to know each other better. Be sure to find out about them during the lunch as well; in fact, it may be prudent to do some research about them or their facility before meeting in person with them. Remember to be yourself! You don't have to do a hard sell, but you do need to appear confident and be able to communicate about your business. Remember to practice with friends or loved ones if necessary. Having lunch is generally a casual time. Be sure to dress

Figure 2.1 Sample brochure.

Families in TRANSITION

Helping individuals, couples and families adjust to family changes

Individuals and families are constantly changing, in transition - passing through a series of life stages. These changes are necessary, but can also be very stressful and painful. FAMILIES IN TRANSITION provides a safe and supportive place to learn, grow, and develop as a person and as a family.

COUNSELING FOR INDIVIDUALS, COUPLES, AND FAMILIES

Therapy is offered to meet your special needs by a caring and experienced Clinical Nurse Specialist. Effective problem-solving, communication, and other inter-personal skills are learned to promote personal growth and healthy relationships. Children, adolescents, and adults of all ages are welcome.

PROVIDING SERVICES FOR:

- Alcoholism/ Substance Abuse
- 12 Step Programs
- Co-Dependency
- Dysfunctional Families/ACOA
- Depression
- Anxiety
- Parent/Child Concerns
- Marriage/Relationship Issues
- Divorce/Re-Marriage
- Eating Disorders - Body Image
- Sexual Difficulties
- Sexual Abuse - Incest/Rape
- Battering/Domestic Violence
- Gay/Lesbian Issues
- Life Crisis/Stress
- Low Self-Esteem
- Job Stress/Unemployment
- Health - Illness Problems

SPECIAL GROUPS/ COUNSELING

Group Counseling
Survivors of sexual abuse, co-dependency, assertiveness training, parenting, step-families, and stress reduction.

Child/Adolescent Counseling

Step-Family Counseling

Single-Parent Counseling

Health Promotion/ Nutrition

Christian/Spiritual
Biblical counseling and spiritual encouragement for those who desire it. An ordained Minister is available for Pastoral counseling.

OFFICE POLICIES

Office hours are Monday through Friday from 8 a.m. to 8 p.m. and are by appointment only. Fees are based upon the clients ability to pay. Insurance billing is available.

Figure 2.1 (continued)

Families in TRANSITION

Helping individuals, couples and families adjust to family changes

Susanne Fine M.A., R.N, C.S. is a licensed Registered Nurse and a certified Psychiatric Mental-Health Clinical Nurse Specialist. She obtained her Master's Degree in Counseling from Lewis & Clark College and has advanced training in Marriage/Family Therapy. She has nearly 15 years experience in Nursing, is a published author, and has taught various seminars in the community and at the university level.

She holds memberships in The California Nurses Association, The American Association for Marriage & Family Therapy, The California Association of Marriage/Family Therapy, and The Claremont Chamber of Commerce.

FOOTHILL

BONITA

219

10 FREEWAY

Please call for an appointment
(909) 626-0163
219 N. Indian Hill Blvd., Suite 201
Claremont, California 91711

(909) 626-0163
219 N. Indian Hill Blvd., Suite 201
Claremont, California 91711

34

```
┌─────────────────────────────────────────────────┐
│                                                   │
│   LOGO                    (555) 555-5555          │
│                                                   │
│                                                   │
│   JANE DOE, M.S., R.N., C.S.                      │
│   Clinical Nurse Specialist                       │
│   Counseling & Consultation                       │
│                                                   │
│                                                   │
│   35 Main St., Suite 101                          │
│   Anywhere, California 99999                      │
│                                                   │
└─────────────────────────────────────────────────┘
```

FIGURE 2.2   Business Card Format.

comfortably and neatly (try a fairly business or professional look), but choose something that you really feel good in. Be sure to bring along extra brochures and business cards to give them if they would like. Then, in the future when you are planning group or special speaking engagements, you can call them or send them a notice as well. The more they hear from you, the more they will remember you. Just don't badger them or seem too eager.

When starting a practice in a new town, it's good to say that you have a small practice and that you're building. After you have some clients, you can say you have a full-time practice, etc. Remember to be humble without being self-effacing. *Believe in yourself and others will too!*

The first few meetings will be the most difficult, so I suggest that you start with someone whom you already know somewhat. If you are coming out of an acute care setting, try to invite the director of nursing or the head of the psychiatric unit or a physician along. Start simple and build up your confidence.

Remember to practice on the phone as well. If you are declined for lunch or breakfast, then be sure to follow up with the materials. Keep an ongoing list of names, numbers, and addresses of your contacts and be sure to date and mark off when you last had contact. Remember to follow up again in three to six months, or anytime that you are speaking or doing a group that may be of interest to them. After my initial marketing, I can usually just work on maintaining contacts who are sending me some clients.

Another helpful hint is to refer some clients to professional sources, but be sure that you can feel confident about their services. I routinely refer to psychiatrists with whom I am very comfortable, so that my clients can have physicals or medication. It is important for you to have a good working relationship with at least one physician, but it doesn't have to be a psychiatrist. If a client doesn't have a regular doctor and needs an antidepressant, or some other medication, it is good to know of a doctor with whom you trust to follow up, and who is supportive of your work.

One of the best ways to develop working relationships with doctors is to contact them when you start to see their patients (after getting written permission from the client). Then, call to inform them of their patient's progress and to ask for feedback, pertinent medical information, and how they may assist you in giving the client the best treatment. The focus should be on the doctor and finding out about his or her practice. You would do well to offer to keep them abreast of changes in your client's care. This may also be done with the client's pastors. It is useful to offer to meet with them in person to get acquainted and to let them know that you would be interested in referring people to them.

Public Speaking

One of the very best ways to get referrals is to do some public speaking or workshops. You may feel very uncomfortable about this, but start with a very small group (fewer than 10) and work your way up. You may never feel comfortable about speaking to a group of 200, but you would be surprised how easy it is to speak to an informal group that you are doing for free. Remember to keep it simple, short, and only present something you really know well. Be sure to make an outline and have notes for yourself. Having hand-outs is also appreciated and you can always fall back on those if you get too nervous. It is essential that you be yourself and let people see who you are. Try to be personable, but professional and friendly. Smile a lot!

If you feel comfortable, and it is appropriate, share something about your own recovery or experiences. What do you have in common with this group? It would be best to start with a group with which you have a lot of interest or experience. Then you will seem more natural and knowledgeable without appearing too clinical. Remember, you're donating your time and most groups will be thrilled to have you speak and are usually *very* grateful. This can be a nice confidence booster.

Formal presentations/workshops or talks to colleagues are different. Here, you need to be more polished and organized, but again, it's important to be yourself. Try to ascertain if your group is familiar with your topic. You don't want to bore them, nor do you want to be beyond their scope either. It is important that you also bring business cards, brochures, and so on to all of your speaking engagements.

Getting to know the other mental-health professionals in your community is important. Try to minimize a competitive approach, rather attempt to convey a professional and firm attitude to your right to practice. There are plenty of people in need of help, especially if you specialize in a particular approach or treatment issue. You will want to let your colleagues know so that they can make some specific referrals to you.

Consultation

Another area that can bring in some referrals for you is direct consultations to other special interest groups or nurse colleagues. There is a specialty called psychiatric liaison nursing that involves a consultative role in acute care settings and agencies where you can use your advanced skills.[2] Writing articles in the local newspaper, journals, or nursing periodicals can also be useful. Don't be afraid to say that you are available for consultations.

Be sure to always charge for your services, unless you specifically want to offer them for free. This includes reports for clients. Most insurance companies will pay for some special reports (see CPT codes in chapter 4). It's acceptable to give away some free services in the beginning, but remember that you want to have a successful business, which means charging and collecting for your services. You may consider charging a higher fee for first-time clients, especially when billing insurance (use CPT code 90801 for assessments as they usually take a longer time). Other therapists have been successful with reducing their first-time visits or discounting their rates to special groups. You are free to be creative; just remember that your goal is also to be successful as a business.

As mentioned in chapter 1, I prefer to have a sliding scale for clients based upon their ability to pay. Many nonprofit agencies will give you the referral when they know that you have a sliding scale and are willing to negotiate with the clients. Clients are sensitive to the attitude that the money is the most important issue; I always try not to have that be a deciding factor. Yet, clients seem to do better when they are paying for their services. Clients may take the therapist and the therapy process for granted and not be as involved when they do not have to pay for services.

I have read in psychologists' and marriage and family therapists' professional ethics code that some services are to be done at no cost or at a reduced fee (pro bono).[3] Our nursing ethics do not mention this; it is a personal choice. Nurses tend to charge too little and give too many services away for free. It is important to understand your own philosophy about fees before starting a practice. One approach is to bill for professional services, but do not make undue effort to collect from people who do not pay, such as, taking them to small claims court or using collection agencies. Uncollected fees may be then considered your ''pro bono'' work. Another approach is to use a sliding scale which bases fees on the client's ability to pay.

Balancing altruism and care for humanity with sound business sense is optimum. Remember that if you do not focus enough on charging for your services, then you may end up back to work at an agency or hospital. (Please review ''Setting Your Fees'' in chapter 3.)

NOTES

1. Beck, C., Rawlins, R., & Williams, S. (1988). *Mental-Health Psychiatric Nursing*. St. Louis, MO: C. V. Mosby.
2. American Nurses Association. (1990). *Standards of Pychiatric Consultation Liaison Nursing Practice*. Washington, DC: Author.
3. Thompson, A. (1983). *Ethical Concerns in Psychotherapy and Their Legal Ramifications*. New York: University Press.

Chapter **3**

FUNDAMENTALS OF STARTING A PRACTICE

There are enormous decisions to be made once you have decided to go into private practice. After you have decided that you want to pursue a private practice, talk with other psychiatric nurses or other mental-health clinicians. It is really great to have a mentor while you are starting out (see nurse support groups). Your master's degree program may not have offered you much advice on the how tos, so you will be going back to school (so-to-speak) to learn about how to succeed in this arena.

For marketing strategies, please review chapter 2. Before you can adequately market yourself, there are a few basics that need to be accomplished. You need to decide whether you want to be in solo practice or with other clinicians, such as nurses, doctors, or other therapists. It may be cost effective to do this at first, and then expand on your own.

START UP

You may work for a while and save money to start up a practice. You may get a small business loan to purchase a practice (contact local banks or the Small Business Administration). If you buy a practice, generally the way to decide what it is worth is to average the net earnings for three years and divide by three. This figure can be the selling price. Otherwise, you may take out a small business loan to start up from scratch—usually

$10,000 will be adequate. Loans or purchase price can also be tax deducted.

OFFICE

You need to find some office space right away. One thing I have done is to rent a suite and sublet one or two of the offices to other mental-health professionals. That helps cover my rent. I continue to work independently to keep expenses down, but I also employ 2–3 other types of therapists, for example, MFCCs, LCSWs or PhDs as independent contractors. My business receives 40% of their income. Both are easy ways to keep expenses down and increase my profit margin. I refer most of my evening work to them and overflow referrals. They also generate clientele.

Try to find office space that is close to where you live if the market of people needing therapy seems to be good. Try to stay away from an office in your home, although I have tried it. Some of the pitfalls in having an office at home are: the lack of personal privacy, the tendency to "live your job," it may decrease a professional image, and it may be a risk hazard with unstable clients. Some positives are: the convenience, lower cost, ease in seeing clients on an emergency basis, or if seeing a few clients scattered throughout the day. It may be helpful to start out in your home until the practice is flourishing, and then transfer to an office outside of your home. My office is only five minutes away which easily accommodates an emergency or weekend session, and it enhances my career satisfaction because I don't have to spend a lot of time driving.

Make sure that you don't have your office in too rural an area. Your clients should have relatively easy access to you from roads, nearby cities, or freeways. Try to pick an office that is not too small; a window is a plus. You must make sure that you have a waiting room that is big enough to accommodate a family, or a number of clients especially if you share space with other therapists. Make sure that you have access to a bathroom as well. It is important to have wheelchair access or access for those with disabilities, too.

Once you have decided on your office, sign the rental or lease agreement only after thorough reading of the contract. Compare offices that include utilities, cleaning, carpet service, and other options with those that do not. Most offices include utilities except for phone, and many include cleaning services, but not all do. Don't hesitate to get an attorney's opinion if you feel it's necessary. Most offices are on a one to three year lease agreement, or you may sublet month to month. You should ask if it is transferable to someone else if you move or sell your practice. Also, find out if you can sublet to others.

WHAT TO CALL YOURSELF

You need to decide if you will have a fictitious name, Doing Business As (DBA), or if you will just go by your name. Fictitious business name refers to having a business that has a logo or title other than your legal name. It is not necessary, and is used mostly when more than one practitioner are in the same group. It also can draw client's attention because of the special name or information contained within. For example, Families in Transition alludes to families that are going through changes. Clients who are experiencing changes, or who want family therapy, likely will be looking under this heading. This is especially true for those who look in the yellow pages of the phone book and who do not have a personal reference to you. One down side is when clients have a referral to you, but do not know your business name. They may have trouble locating you unless you are listed with both the fictitious business name and your own together.

A logo usually costs a few hundred dollars to have a graphic artist design, or costs nothing if you just use your own name or design your own logo. New computer programs have graphic capabilities as an option. It is strictly a personal decision.

If you decide on a fictitious Name, such as Families in Transition, you need to file it with a local newspaper, who then files it with the county recorder's office. It must be reprinted/renewed approximately every 4–5 years. It will be printed in the paper for a period of time, usually three to five weeks. There is a special area in the newspaper (business section) especially for this purpose. This is absolutely necessary by law. After doing this, go to your local Chamber of Commerce/City Hall to apply for a business license—before starting to see clients. You will need a copy of the fictitious business filing for them as well. The fees are based upon income, but are usually between $50.00 and $150.00 a year. They will give you a temporary business license, which you must post on public display at your office. Remember to post the final one as well.

You will also need your business license when getting a business checking account. You can open up a business savings for as little as $300 (minimum balance) or for free, but the problem with a business account is that at some banks you need to keep a minimum balance greater than $5,000. Check with your bank about this. If you do not have a business account, make sure that clients make the checks out to you. You may run all of your money through your personal checking account as long as you keep good records. I have a business account for when I get checks made out to my business name. The bank will not often deposit a check made out to your business into your personal checking account.

Next, look into office insurance. This is very inexpensive, but will really save you if someone trips on the rug, you have a fire, or some other mishap. If you plan to have employees, then you must have special insurance to cover them. Most policies don't cover subletees, so be sure to tell your tenants that they need to have their own. If you sublet, be sure to have a rental agreement with a 30- or 60-day notice for changes in the rental agreement or vacating of the premises for both you and them. This will allow you enough time to find someone else. Also, be sure that they know that they cannot use your name or the name of the business. Make sure they have current licenses and malpractice insurance. Rental forms can be found in most stationery stores.

You need to furnish your office with furniture that is appealing and professional looking. Try to have soft, muted tones and furniture that provides warmth. You will be spending a lot of time in this place, so be sure that it is something that you like. If decorating is not one of your strong points, you may want to consider hiring a decorator. Try to keep the cost down, but don't buy cheap looking or poorly made items. You might want to join a wholesale club and buy at a discount once you have a business license.

A desk and a lockable filing cabinet for your charts are essential (the latter dictated by law). A long couch that can accommodate four people is nice, along with at least two chairs. Can you accommodate families or not? Families may not want to sit together on a couch, so there need to be plenty of options. Be sure to get *yourself* a really nice, stuffed, comfortable chair; since you will be spending many hours in it, make sure it is comfortable.

EQUIPMENT

Having a computer with a laser printer can save you enormous time and money. You can have your billing and forms on disk, and computers. These can be written off on your taxes as supplies/business expenses. I prefer IBM compatible machines, although Macintosh computers are fine also. Both types run billing and word processing software (i.e., WordPerfect). It is important to have a hard drive with enough storage space (memory). Try to get some information from others that are knowledgeable about computers. There are many computer and software options, and it is beyond the scope of this book to describe them. Try your library as well, for books and magazines on the subject. Doing research on your equipment is essential. For my IBM compatible computer, I prefer WordPerfect for word processing, a business software called QuickBooks or Money, and do my billing on LotusWorks.

SUPPLIES

Besides buying basic office supplies, such as a stapler, pens, paper, and so on, you will need a phone that allows you to put the caller on "hold." I find "call waiting" useful as well. Fax and copy machines are optional. Their costs can be prohibitive unless you have great use for them, although some lower-cost models are now available for the "home office." It is probably best to wait for these until you are really well established. Do buy yourself a nice leather appointment book; one that has replaceable calendars with phone numbers in the back is best. You may need to call clients after hours and while away from the office, so it is good to have a handy place for that information.

After furnishing your office and waiting room, and getting office supplies, you are ready for the next step—brochures, business cards, and stationery. Go to a copy center nearby and find out about prices for these items. Try to design your own (see pages 33–35 for samples), but if you can't, hire someone to do it.

It is probably best to order about 500 business cards, 100 brochures, and 250 envelopes and letterhead to start. This way, you can keep costs down and be sure to have plenty on hand for workshops, and so on. Try to hand out your cards and brochures to as many people as you can (see marketing, chapter 3). Choose a color (or colors) that you like and that reflects your style.

When designing your brochures and business cards, try to collect at least six examples from other therapists or agencies. Then, play around with some ideas on paper, or on your computer. What kind of counseling do you offer? What populations are you targeting? Do you want a twofold or trifold brochure? A copy center can typeset it for a very low price, and the brochures can be copied onto nice paper rather than being printed. This will save money, but doesn't cut down on the quality.

Be sure to have an explanation of who you are so people can get to know your unique qualifications. A nice touch is to add the organizations that you belong to or publications you have written. Remember that this is a powerful marketing tool and needs to be professional looking.

Be aware of any advertising guidelines from your state Board of Nursing. For example, California currently dictates that we cannot use the terms "Psychotherapy" or "Psychotherapist," even though they are in our Standards of Practice.[1] It is unlawful to make false or misleading statements and this is considered a misdemeanor. The California Board of Behavioral Science Examiners specifies that marriage, family and child counselors (MFCC) must have a license number printed on all materials. You need to be very careful, especially in states like California where there are so many MFCCs and other competitive practitioners. I do know of some nurses who use the term Psychotherapy in California, but I personally do not. In many states, it seems to be in common usage without a problem. Other terms that can be used are: therapist, nurse therapist, psychiatric nurse, CNS, counselor, nurse consultant, and nurse counselor.

RECORD KEEPING AND FORMS

In order to start seeing clients, you need to have some forms put together to make a chart. There are many ways to set up charts; some samples are included here. These can be adapted for your personal use, but don't be afraid to devise your own to meet your special needs.

I usually put my charts in manila file folders with various tab positions that I write the individual client's name on. Some agencies assign the files numbers; it's up to you. I fasten the papers with a two-hole #22 metal fastener, because I like to keep the files neat. My files are in alphabetical order in my locked file cabinet.

All of the identifying information goes on the bottom, and the notes are on the top. I add notes as needed. The statement form is unattached in the files so that I can pull it out for ease of billing. Having all the forms and a billing system on computer will save you incredible amounts of time—and time is money! You may want to photocopy the forms in quantity to keep on hand.

Client–Therapist Relationship Form

The Client–Therapist Relationship form is one of the most important. Some states require therapists to have this form, but even if your state

TABLE 3.1   The Client–Therapist Relationship

All clients are requested to read and agree to the following statements as a condition of initiating counseling services.

CONFIDENTIALITY

1. All information and material discussed within the context of the therapeutic setting shall be held in strict confidence by the therapist *except* if any of the following should occur:
   a. Therapist believes client to be a danger to self.
   b. Therapist believes client to be a danger to others.
   c. Therapist believes client to be gravely disabled and unable to adequately care for him/herself.
   d. Therapist believes a child (or and elder) is being abused.

   In the event of any of these exceptions, the therapist has a moral/ethical/legal duty to break the client's confidence in order to intervene appropriately.
2. In the event that the therapist needs to obtain additional information or to discuss aspects of the client's case with other professionals or agencies, the client will be asked to sign a RELEASE OF INFORMATION, giving permission to obtain written or verbal information.
3. If the client is a minor child, (s)he is entitled to the same confidentiality as an adult, however, parental consultation is available to discuss case progress. The parent(s) may also be asked to participate in any or all of the child's counseling sessions.
4. Client agrees not to solicit the therapist in an adversarial support dispute, nor will client attempt to subpoena the therapist's records for the same.

RESPONSIBILITY FOR TREATMENT

1. Client understands that the therapist makes no claims for success of treatment. Responsibility for responding to and implementing therapeutic interventions and homework assignments rests solely with the *individual* client, even though there may be more than one person involved in the therapy sessions.
2. If the client becomes dissatisfied with the treatment process, (s)he agrees to express the discontent *in the therapy session* where the potential for resolution or appropriate referral or termination exists.
3. Client assumes the responsibility for attending all scheduled appointments on time. Sessions are 50–60 minutes in length.
4. If it becomes necessary to miss an appointment, the client agrees to cancel at least 24 hours in advance of the scheduled time, or be charged the usual fee.

(Continued)

5. In the event of an emergency, please try to contact your therapist. If unable to reach your therapist, please contact your personal physician, or the nearest police or sheriff, or go to your nearest hospital emergency room.

FINANCIAL RESPONSIBILITY

1. Client and therapist have agreed to a fee of \$_____ per session.

2. Client agrees to pay at each session. There will be no balance due carried over from one session to the next. Client also agrees to pay for each session missed, unless cancelled at least 24 hours in advance. Insurance companies will not be billed for missed appointments or late cancellations.

3. The therapist agrees to file insurance claims with the client's insurance carrier, if applicable, so that the client can be reimbursed for expenses incurred. Client is ultimately responsible for the total bill, even in the event that the insurance claim is denied.

I/we have read and agree to the above statements and indicate my/our understanding and agreement by signing below.

_____   _____
(Signature of Client)   (Date)

_____   _____
(Signature of Client)   (Date)

_____   _____
(Signature of Therapist)   (Date)

does not, it is prudent to use it anyway. It makes sure that you cover some essential legal aspects with the client, such as confidentiality.[2] It also serves as a signed, written document that they understand the terms of therapy, including fees. See Table 3.1 for an example of this document.

If the bill is disputed, or a court case arises, the document can be presented to show that it was signed by the client. Therapy is a contract; you have an ethical and legal responsibility to the client.

Confidential Admissions Data Form

This is also one of the most important forms because it is a record of important client information, including insurance information necessary for billing (see Table 3.2). Should the client refuse to pay or ''disappears,'' you have some information to help in collection. Most collection agencies

TABLE 3.2   Confidential Admissions Data

NAME:_____DATE:_____

DATE OF BIRTH:_____SS#:_____EDUCATION:_____

ADDRESS:_____
                              (Number)   (Street)

_____
              (City)   (State)   (Zip)

PHONE:(_____)_____(_____)_____

AGE:_____EMPLOYER_____OCCUPATION:_____

May I call you at work? yes_____no_____

MONTHLY INCOME:_____MARITAL STATUS:_____

HOW LONG:_____NAME OF SPOUSE:_____

AGE:_____OCCUPATION:_____EMPLOYER:_____

NAME OF CHILDREN:_____AGE:_____IN HOME?_____

_____   _____   _____

_____   _____   _____

_____   _____   _____

_____   _____   _____

RELIGION:_____REFERRAL SOURCE:_____

May I send a thank-you note to your referral source?_____

FAMILY DOCTOR:_____
                              (Name)   (Address)

INSURANCE INFORMATION:

Name of insurance company:_____

Address:_____

Phone number - (800) if possible:_____

Name of policy holder/insured:_____

His/her social security/ID#:_____

Employer name:_____

Who is covered under this plan?_____

Policy#:_____

Group#:_____

Table 3.2 *(Continued)*

Do you have coverage for out-patient psychiatric or mental health care?_____What are the reimbursement schedules?_____

Deductible per year:_____Is it met for this year?_____

NAME OF CLOSEST RELATIVE:_____

ADDRESS:_____PHONE:_____

PLEASE LIST ANY DIFFICULTIES YOU ARE NOW EXPERIENCING:

_____

_____

_____

_____

HAVE YOU EVER HAD COUNSELING BEFORE? YES_____NO_____

IF YES, WITH WHOM, WHERE, WHEN, AND FOR WHAT REASON?

_____

_____

_____

PLEASE EXPLAIN WHY YOU ARE SEEKING COUNSELING NOW?

_____

_____

_____

WHAT WOULD YOU LIKE TO SEE HAPPEN AS A RESULT OF THERAPY?

_____

_____

_____

_____

_____

charge a small percentage of actual monies collected. Most people don't like to fill out forms, but it is important to have at least their address, phone numbers, and social security number. As mentioned previously, I also keep client phone numbers in the back of my appointment book in case I need to reach them after hours or at home. Encourage your clients to come in 5 to 10 minutes before their first session to fill out the forms so that the whole session can be used for therapy.

I put the Client–Therapist Agreement and the Admissions Data forms on a clipboard along with a brochure, business card, and a pen.

Intake Form

Many therapists in private practice do not have a formal intake form; it is more common in agencies. Yet, I find it very useful to place the presenting problem in the context of the client's personal and family history. It is a valuable reference point, even through therapy may take a quite different turn (see Table 3.3). Initially, I also like to get a medical, drug/alcohol history, and to complete a three-generation genogram. A genogram is a specialized family history that looks at family lineage, likened to a family tree (Table 3.4, p. 52). In the context of therapy, the therapist looks beyond this to patterns of abuse, relationship dysfunctions, medical problems, and family secrets or rules that negatively affect the client today. This extensive family history is incredibly worthwhile. It tells so much about the client and why he/she is having the particular presenting problem. For a good beginning primer on genograms see *Genograms in Family Assessment.*[3]

I also think that it is a good idea to be familiar enough with both nursing diagnosis and DSM IV diagnosis styles so that you write them in even if you don't bill insurance. Not practicing them may cause your skills to deteriorate.

Mental Status Exam Form

This is also an optional part of the assessment. Although you may do one spontaneously in your head, you may not realize how easy it is to fill one of these out. I use them on my more seriously disturbed clients, and always if there is any doubt about psychosis. Remember that more seriously disturbed, psychotic, or suicidal patients should be referred to a psychiatrist. It is good to document the mental status exam any time that your client is decompensating for any reason.

I often use the Beck Depression Inventory to assess for the seriousness of depression and to evaluate suicidal ideation more thoroughly. This

TABLE 3.3   Intake

DATE:_____CLIENT NAME:_____

PRESENTING PROBLEM:

_____
_____
_____
_____
_____
_____
_____
_____
_____
_____
_____
_____
_____
_____
_____
_____
_____
_____
_____

MEDICAL HISTORY:

_____
_____
_____
_____
_____
_____
_____

MEDICATION:

_____
_____
_____
_____
_____
_____

DRUG/ALCOHOL USAGE:

_____
_____
_____
_____
_____

TABLE 3.3 *(Continued)*

FAMILY HISTORY:

_____

_____

_____

_____

_____

_____

NURSING DIAGNOSIS:

_____

_____

_____

_____

_____

_____

_____

GOALS:

_____

_____

_____

_____

_____

DIAGNOSTIC IMPRESSION: (DSM IV)

AXIS I_____

AXIS II_____

AXIS III_____

AXIS IV_____

AXIS V_____

(GAF)_____

helps me to determine if the patient needs to be placed on antidepressants, and to further evaluate any suicidal ideation. This can be used many times during the course of treatment.

TABLE 3.4   Three Generation Genogram

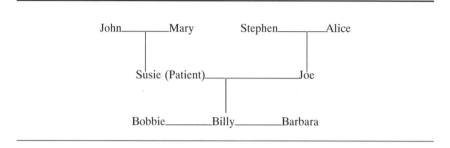

Release of Information TO and FROM Forms

These two Release of Information forms may be combined for ease of use. It is mandatory that before you talk with *anyone* about the client, that you have a signed "Release of Information" first. Of course, if it meets the criteria for breaking confidentiality, then this isn't necessary (see Client–Therapist Relationship). I always like to have the client sign one—even after the fact. Remember that you need one to bill, and talk to insurance companies or managed care case workers, too. Get in the habit of having them sign one up front. (See Table 3.5.)

Notes Form

Notes can be written up on a printed form or on any piece of lined paper or legal pad (Table 3.6). Begin with the date and the session number—#1, 2, and so on. You should write in black ink in case you need to photocopy them. Notes should contain all of the pertinent information about the session: client affect, interventions, responses to treatment, relevant themes, diagnostic impressions, important symptomatology, history, and also the homework assignment. Be brief and succinct; remember that the notes may be subpoenaed in the future.

It isn't necessary to make really detailed notes unless the client is severely ill, suicidal, depressed, or has some other serious condition. Then, I think you should be very detailed and accurate in your accounts. If a client is depressed, chart about suicidal ideation or danger to self/others. Include a mental status check. Don't forget to chart phone conversations that are made after hours or on weekends. Don't forget to chart these

TABLE 3.5   Release of Information

I hereby request and authorize

_____

(therapist)

Name of Counseling Center
Address
City, State, Zip Code

to release or discuss any pertinent information concerning the treatment of

_____   _____

(name)   (date of birth)

to:

_____

(therapist/school/agency)

_____

(address)

_____

(city)   (state)   (zip)

_____   _____

(signature of client or guardian)   (date)

(This authorization shall remain in effect for 60 days or until it is revoked by the client.)

---

conversations with relevant others, such as family or doctor. I sometimes chart who I spoke with and the date or important information when I talk with the insurance company. I review my notes from the previous week before seeing the client. I also sign my notes, but that may be a holdover from hospital nursing.

Statement Form

This form is important to fill out with the relevant insurance information in as much detail as possible. I also like to have the contact person/case manager name and 800 numbers to call. I usually include the reimbursement schedule, address of where to send the claims, and other important client information (see Table 3.7, Statement Form). This form is taken

TABLE 3.6   Client Notes

Date	Number and Type of Contact	Notes

out of the chart to do insurance billing. It is helpful to keep a per/session account of what you charge, what the client pays, and what insurance payments are made. This way you know what the client's balance is at all times. Try to have cash-paying clients pay as they go and not build up an outstanding balance.

TABLE 3.7   Statement Form

Name Insured_____Name Client_____

DOB_____Insured SS#_____PH#_____

Address_____Employer_____

_____Referral_____

Insurance_____PH#_____

Address_____Fee:_____

_____GRP or EID#_____

Benefits_____Deductible_____

Contact Person_____PH#_____

DX1_____2_____3_____4_____5_____

DATE	DEBIT	CREDIT	BAL. DUE		DATE	DEBIT	CREDIT	BAL. DUE

It is advisable to have the clients with insurance pay the co-payment (what the insurance won't pay) at the time of each visit (i.e., 20% to 50%). Some therapists have the client pay the full fee and then have them

TABLE 3.8 Physician's Referral

Dear Doctor_____:

Your patient,_____

DOB_____, has come to us for counseling services. We would like a referral from you stating that it is alright with you for (s)he to get therapy from us. Please sign the following and return to us at your earliest convenience. We will keep you informed of their progress as need be.

Sincerely,

_____

Agency/Therapist signature

_____
_____
_____
_____

(Name and Address of Agency)

....

I am referring_____DOB_____,
to Name of Agency/Therapist for counseling services.

_____   _____

(Doctor's signature)   (Date)

_____
_____
_____
_____

(Name and Address)

_____

collect directly from their insurance company. This is ideal, but most people can't afford to do this. The more you can collect your monies up front, the more successful you will be.

Physician's Referral Form

This form can be mailed or given to the client's doctor in advance of seeing the client—if possible—or as soon after. You don't need to send it to the insurance company, although some will ask for a copy. It is

TABLE 3.9   Financial Agreement

I/we have agreed to be responsible for a fee of $_____ per session. I/we are proposing to pay $_____ per session (_____% of the fee) and to assign insurance benefits for payment of $_____ per session (_____% of the fee). I/we realize that irrespective of whether the insurance carrier pays or not, responsibility for the payment rests with me/ us. If at any time my/our financial situation or insurance coverage changes, I/we agree to inform the therapist and to discuss the renegotiation of this agreement.

(Client)	(Date)
(Client)	(Date)
(Therapist)	(Date)

useful to keep it in the chart for reference. Again, remember that some insurance companies require a doctor's referral, so always try to get one. Be sure to put the doctor's name as a referral on the bill, or you may be denied a claim for failing to get one. It is good to keep the physician informed that their client is in counseling. This also serves as a marketing tool. See Table 3.8 for an example.

Financial Agreement Form

This is an optional form and is included here in case you change your original financial agreement (Table 3.9). This keeps both you and your client accountable in case of misunderstandings.

Weekly Summary Experience Log Form

It is a good idea to keep track of your total monthly or yearly hours of experience for the first two years, especially if you are just starting out. Try to keep track of how many individual versus family (includes children) therapy that you do. Remember to include any type of supervision hours, even peer supervision. This form can also be used in getting your Clinical Nurse Specialist Supervised experience. The ANCC (American Nurses

TABLE 3.10   Weekly Summary Experience Log

Date_____ Name_____
Work Setting_____

Week of:										Total Hours
Couples, Family or Child Therapy										
Individual Therapy										
Group Therapy										
Telephone Counseling										
Individual Supervision										
Group Supervision										
Workshops, Conferences, etc.										
Writing Reports, Progress Notes										
Total for Week										

Name of Supervisor:_____
Title/Certification:_____
Supervisor Signature:_____
Total Hours This Period:_____

Credentialing Center) doesn't require it, but it is easier to keep track of your hours this way, and also serves as permanent record (Table 3.10).

Permission to Audio/Videotape Record Form

If you are doing any recording or audiotaping for school or supervision, please be sure to have the client give you permission by signing this

TABLE 3.11   Permission for Audio/Videotape Recording

I/we have been informed that on occasion my/our therapy sessions will be audio and/or video recorded. I/we understand that the purpose of the recording is to facilitate the therapeutic process and that the recorded material will be reviewed only for educational or supervisorial purposes and will thereafter be erased.

(client)   (client)

(therapist)   (date)

TABLE 3.12   Accounts Receivable Ledger

	MONTH OF:			
NAME OF CLIENT	2/1-2/7	2/8-2/14	2/15-2/21	2/22-2/28
DOE, J	100-	100-	100-	
FRIEND, K	75-	300-	75-	25-
JONES, A	50-	50-	50-	250-
WIDOW, M	100-	100-	100-	100-
TOTAL	325-	550-	225-	475-

TOTAL FOR MONTH = $1,575.00

form (Table 3.11). It assures confidentiality and shows that they are in agreement. It can be very helpful to see yourself in session and get feedback from a colleague or supervisor to help improve your skills.

Ledgers—Accounts Receivable Form

It is essential that you have complete and accurate ledgers of your accounts in case you ever get audited, and for ease in preparing your taxes. (Tax information will be covered later.) You can use pre-printed ledger books, but there are many different systems out there. (A sample of Accounts Receivable Form is shown in Table 3.12.) Go to a large well-stocked office supply store and browse through all of their accounting materials.

As indicated on the forms, write in the client's last name *in pencil* followed by the amount received at each session. I also add the insurance or other payments I receive as well. Add up weekly columns at the end of the month for a monthly total income. The amount for each week is totalled at the bottom and circled with the date of the bank deposit. All of the deposit slips are kept and attached to the back of each ledger. At the end of the month, I take them out of the book and place them in a large envelope marked for the year to keep as a permanent record. Then, when I do my taxes, I take out the ledgers and add them up for a total of earnings for that year. Having it written in a form that is easily checked is a smart way to do business. I give clients receipts for cash or checks only if they request one. A receipt book is kept handy in my drawer. If a client wants a copy of a regular bill, I run one off from the computer. I have had an account balance questioned by a client only once.

Remember, your statement forms have the payments on them as well. This system has some checks and balances and literally takes a few minutes a month to do. You can adapt it for your own special use.

Ledgers—Accounts Payable Form

Just like the accounts receivable ledger, this one is also filled out on a monthly basis in pencil (Table 3.13). Each week, I write in who I paid, for what, and the amount. Each week, *in pencil*, total the expenses and add them up at the end of the month. Then when it is time to do taxes, it is easy to see what has been paid for tax-deductible items (see tax information below). All of my receipts are kept and are attached to each monthly ledger for a permanent record.

It really is easy and quick to keep good records. Don't let yourself get sloppy. Once you are in the habit of doing this, it will be effortless for you. There is no reason that you can't do your own taxes, especially if you consult a tax consultant or CPA first.

These are most of the forms that you will need and examples will follow. The billing and financially related forms are at the end of chapter 4.

TAX INFORMATION

Since you are self-employed, you will be paying quite a bit for taxes. Therefore, it is imperative that you deduct as many items as you can for tax purposes. I recommend that you consult with a tax accountant prior to starting your business for specific advice or whenever you have questions.

TABLE 3.13   Accounts Receivable Ledger-1993

		MONTH OF:			
DATE	TO WHOM? FOR WHAT	2/1-2/7	2/8-2/14	2/15-2/21	2/22-2/28
2/1	POSTAGE/POST OFF.	12.50			
2/4	COPIES/COPY CTR	2.90			
2/7	FAX/VILLAGE POST	7.00			
2/8	ASSOC. MEMBRSP		75.00		
2/10	BRN-LICENSE REN.		30.00		
2/12	COPIES/COPY CTR		2.00		
2/16	COPIES/COPY CTR			1.45	
2/15	RENT/OWNER			745.00	
2/15	BOOKS/BOOKSTORE			39.59	
2/22	INS. CO./INSURANCE				120.00
2/24	STATIONARY STORE/ SUPPLIES				68.97
2/28	PRINTING/COPY CTR				39.00
TOTAL		22.40	107.00	786.04	227.97

TOTAL FOR MONTH = $1,143.41

The best FREE guide that I have found for tax information for small businesses is: *Tax Guide for Small Business*, Department of Treasury, Internal Revenue Service Publication #334. You may receive it by contacting your local IRS and they will send you one. They may be contacted by phone; call information for a listing or look in the phone book under United States Government Listings.

You can bill under your own social security number, or if you have employees, then you must apply for an Employer Identification Number (unless you hire independent contractors). Insurance companies will send a 1099 (Miscellaneous Earnings) to the IRS for your yearly earnings and you will receive one as well. You don't have to attach these to your tax returns, but do keep them. Remember, if you do any independent contracting for an agency or provider, you must have them give you a 1099 form at the end of the year. If you hire other therapists as independent contractors, then you must also provide them a 1099 tax form for the tax year (due to them by January 31st following the tax year end). Call your local IRS for free 1099s.

The following items are tax deductible, which means that you can deduct them from your earnings so that you pay less taxes. You will need to file both state and federal taxes if you meet the income requirements (please check with your local Internal Revenue Service for state and federal requirements). Ask an accountant about making estimated tax payments on a quarterly basis so that you won't owe a huge amount in April. Tax deductible items:

All Supplies—stamps, paper, cups, photocopying or printing expenses, etc.

Equipment—computers, copier, microwave, furniture, answering machine or service, etc.

Tax Preparation—if you use an accountant

Legal fees/consultations with experts

Books/Journals—''This book''

Membership dues—professional, chamber of commerce, discount warehouse, etc.

Licensing fees

Continuing education to keep up your license and skills (including lodging and meal expenses)

Educational expenses if they are not to change professions, but only to upgrade your skills or help you keep the same job

Travel expenses—if they are part of your job—but not to and from work

Luncheons/food costs—when business-related (only 50% is written off)

Rent/lease expenses—if you sublet, then you must count that as income even though all of it is a deduction

Utilities—even part of the phone bill at home if used for business

Purchase of the business

Insurance for office

Marketing, advertisements—brochures, business cards, yellow pages, etc.

Business license, cost of lease, etc.

Uniforms if used, special clothing

Medical Insurance premiums if you are self-employed

These are the main tax deductible items that you need to be aware of, and it will help you immensely to keep good records with receipts. It really isn't so hard once you get in the habit. Always ask for receipts wherever you go. Again, I like to attach them to the ledger so they are kept neat and easily found if necessary.

SETTING UP

Now you have all that you need to open your doors and set up shop. Decide what kind of schedule you want. Do you want to see a maximum number of clients a day? Do you want to work evenings or weekends? Try to set a schedule that will keep you from being "burned out." My clients are generally working, so they like early morning or afternoon appointments. I do see some people at noon, but usually between noon and two o'clock is empty, so I take my lunch then and rest. Personally, I like to see five to six clients a day. When I see eight a day, I start to feel stressed. You also need to decide if you will see clients for 45 minutes or an hour. Most therapists use the 45-minute routine, but many clients dislike it and are disappointed. I think it's too short, but you need to decide what is best for you. I see clients for 55 to 60 minutes. I do my charting and return phone calls later, at the end of the day. If you do use 45-minute sessions, you can use the last 10 minutes of the hour for charting, relaxation, or for returning phone calls.

Remember, you will spend about 15 minutes a week for every client with your work, charting, and other paperwork. Try to allow an hour a week for follow-up with insurance companies. Remember to be consistent with timing your sessions; do not be late or go over. Good time boundaries are part of the therapeutic process. Twenty hours of direct client contact is considered full-time. It is difficult to do 40 hours a week; it will lead to burnout. This is intense work, pace yourself. You may think that 20 clients a week sounds easy. Once you get there, you'll be surprised how steady it is, and you'll start to relish a missed or cancelled appointment. I see 20–25 clients a week.

I work one or two evenings a week, but most therapists work one to three evenings per week, so I refer my extra evening work to my employees. I do think it is good to work some evenings and an occasional Saturday. It will really be dictated a lot by when your clients are able to come in. It is a good idea to give clients the same time each week for ease of scheduling for yourself and the client. Once you are doing this work, then you can always change your schedule. That's the beauty of your own practice.

It's a good idea to have a sign advertising your business on the door and/or building. Post your business hours as well, unless you think that your hours will be changing often. Your general hours should be on your brochures also.

FEE SCHEDULES

Now let's talk about your fees. What are you going to charge? You need to have a competitive price, without undercharging. The national average for master's-prepared therapists is $70.00 per session, with a range of $30.00 to $120.00.[4] Psychologists (PhDs) make from $70 to $140 per session; their average is about $95. It is possible to make $75,000+ per year if one sees 20 clients a week at an average of $70 per session.

I have a sliding scale fee schedule based on the client's ability to pay (range is $60–$110). People appreciate it when you are willing to negotiate your fees. However, most therapists have a set fee and stick with it. They may have to turn people away who can't afford it. I normally charge my full fee when people have insurance, and lower it for those with less income and no insurance. It is not illegal to discount your fees for cash-paying clients. My average works out to be about $80 per session. If you don't want to work much with insurance companies, your fees can be reduced since clients will be paying cash and not benefiting from insurance. This is a personal decision. Also, some nonprofit agencies that may send you referrals like it if you are willing to charge less for certain clients, such as battered women or lower income clients. Again, it depends on what kind of client you want to work with. Are they unemployed or working? Do they have insurance or not? Try to take these issues into account, along with the client's gross monthly earnings, number of children, and so on. Make a chart to use. A flexible attitude is welcomed by clients.

Too often I have found that nurses charge too little for their services. I have nine years of college, and although I qualify to sit for the MFCC exam, I choose not to even though I have a lot more experience and education than many MFCCs and LCSWs. We as nurses have a wealth of information and experience to draw from. We have built on years of nursing and medical training, unlike most master-level clinicians who have just started seeing clients in their master's programs. Again, you've got to believe in yourself.

Remember also, that you are only going to be working 20+ client contact hours a week, not 40, so you need to adjust for this. Plan on about five extra hours for administrative work at the most. There are a lot of pay-offs to working in a private practice. You can have a flexible schedule and hours, and you don't have to work full-time. Don't get discouraged. They say it takes a year to build a small business and start making money. The more time that you spend marketing, the faster you will have 20 clients a week. I have been able to build a full-time practice in about six months' time.

While your practice is being built up, you may want to keep a part-time nursing job or take out a loan. It's very good if you can buy into an existing practice or if you can apprentice with someone. If you work at an agency and leave, the clients are free to come with you. No one owns the clients, but you should not coerce them or bribe them to come with you. It's their choice. The agency may tell you that the clients must stay with them. Unless you signed a waiver against this or a contract saying that you would not take clients with you when you leave, then the clients are free to see you in your new location. I would not recommend that you sign any such agreement; it may violate fair trade and client's rights. Most people will want to stay with their therapist and are willing to follow him or her. However, if you move too far away, you may lose them. Where I live, there are two valleys separated by a big hill, and even though it is only a few miles apart, clients do not want to travel to the other valley. So think before you put up shop as to where your clients will be coming from geographically.

Ask yourself where you do your shopping, and where you go to the doctor or dentist. Clients may think the same as you do. Watch out for natural boundaries, like the hill I mentioned, and easy access on freeways. Be aware also that if two or more PMHNs get together to determine prices, it is considered price-fixing and is illegal. Also, you cannot give any money to your referral sources for their referrals; that is called kick-backs and is also illegal. If you give out referrals, it is a good idea to give clients a couple of names of people whom you know personally and can trust to be good clinicians. Ask for feedback if they do see someone that you have recommended.

It's important to realize that when you are starting a practice, it will take an investment in time as well as money. You may have to spend at least 10 hours a week to do your marketing at first, but remember that whatever energy you put into it, the rewards are yours. Take pride in what you do to create your own business.

NOTES

1. American Nurses Association. (1982). *Standards of psychiatric-mental health nursing*, VA-F. Washington, DC: Author.
2. Thompson, A. (1983). *Ethical concerns in psychotherapy and their legal ramifications*. New York: University Press.
3. McGoldrick, M., & Gerson, R., (1985). *Genograms in family assessment*. New York: Norton & Co.
4. Ridgewood Financial Institute. (1992). *Psychotherapy finances*. Florida: Author.

Chapter **4**

THIRD-PARTY REIMBURSEMENT

This is one of the most important, and sometimes complicated, but necessary parts of having a private practice. Without third-party reimbursement, it will be difficult to succeed very well. Some therapists do practice without taking insurance assignment, but the potential for expanding their practice is limited. If you exclude managed care as well, then your practice will be severely hampered.

The American Nurses Association (ANA) is providing free (to State Nurse Association [SNA] Members) consultation for direct reimbursement.[1] Call the ANA at (202) 554-4444, ext. 446 or ext. 282 to schedule your appointment. Non-SNA members will be charged $110.00 per half-hour; Visa and Mastercard are accepted.

First, you need to know about the different categories of insurance and the specific state and federal laws that govern insurance compensation, which is sometimes referred to as vendorship. Next, you need to be able to work with insurance companies about reimbursing your services directly. To do this, you must be aware of your right to practice (see chapter 1), and also have a professional billing process that will expedite your payments.

When contacting an insurance company or managed care company, do so as soon after the client contacts you as possible, and preferably before actually seeing them. Make sure that you have the client's ID# (social security number), name of the insured, birthdate, employer, and group number if applicable. Ask the insurance company what the deductible is and if they have met it for the year. Many clients say they have met the deductible, but haven't. Always assume that the deductible is not met until processed by the insurance company. If the deductible has not been met, or is only partially met, then the sessions must be paid for by the client directly to the therapist until the dollar amount is reached. Do send in a bill though, as the insurance company will not credit the fees for service and count them towards the deductible until they receive a bill from the provider. For example: the client has a $200.00 per year deductible. It is the first part of the calendar year and so none of it has been met. The charges for therapy are $100.00 per session. The client will need to pay the first two sessions ($200) to the therapist; after that, they may begin to pay the co-payment amount and the therapist will collect the balance from the insurance company. For a client whose insurance company pays 50%, the client would pay the therapist $50.00 starting with the third visit and for all subsequent visits for the rest of the calendar year, or until the maximum benefits have been reached. This is assuming that the therapist is willing to bill the insurance company for the balance. Deductibles are irrelevant when collecting the full fees from the client and billing so that the client will be reimbursed directly from their insurance company. Many managed care companies do not have a deductible for mental-health services.

Then, you need to ask who is covered under the plan, how many sessions or what maximum dollar amount is allowable per year, how much they will actually pay per session (and maximum fee they will consider per session), and also what kind of providers are listed. If they say any licensed provider, then that is the best. Most typically, they will say MD, PhD, MFCC, and LCSW. You can ask about nurses, but many won't know. Usually, if a master's-prepared provider is listed, it will be fairly easy to get reimbursement. You will have a harder time if they limit it to PhDs and MDs only, depending on the type of insurance (see below). Don't be afraid to call Provider Relationships to find out if advanced practice nurses are covered. Refer to the sample letters about how to challenge their decisions if turned down (Tables 4.1–4.3).

One resource cited the following states as mandating some form of third-party coverage for Advanced Practice Nurses.[2]

Alaska	Maine	New Mexico
Arizona	Maryland	New York
California	Massachusetts	North Dakota
Colorado	Minnesota	Pennsylvania
Connecticut	Mississippi	South Dakota
Delaware	Montana	Utah
Florida	Nevada	Washington
Iowa	New Hampshire	West Virginia
Kansas	New Jersey	

TABLE 4.1   Letter for Denial of Claims by Self-Insured Companies

Client's Name
Address
Phone Number

(This is for writing to Self-Insured Companies and can be adapted for other insurance companies)
Date
(Insurance Company name and address)
Re: Denial of claims
Group #
SS#
Dear Claims Reviewer:
I am responding to your letter which denies payment for my out-patient mental health services received from **(name of therapist and agency name)**. It seems that you are denying my claims based on the fact that I am seeing a clinical nurse specialist as my therapist which you say that you do not recognize as an approved provider.

I am aware that the **(Name of Insurance)** plan is governed by federal law (ERISA) because it is a self-insured welfare benefit plan. It seems that you are taking the position that federal law preempts state law, and that you feel that you are not bound by (add State Insurance codes here) California's Freedom of Choice laws (see California Insurance Codes 10177 and 10177.8) and thereby limit the providers from which I may select for the benefits that *are* covered under my plan. (Please insert your particular state's insurance codes here.)

I feel that I am making progress seeing this nurse-therapist and I don't want to change to another mental health provider because of some rule or policy that does not recognize the fact that this provider is licensed and qualified to provide counseling services under state law. It seems that the intent of my plan would be to obtain quality medical services, not to limit the accessibility to them especially if it would not change my benefits or cost to you. In addition, I don't think that this is unreasonable.

Since out-patient counseling services are provided through my plan, I don't understand why you have limited my freedom to choose the provider of my choice. Seeing a psychologist or psychiatrist would only be more expensive to you, and may not meet my needs as well.

It seems that the intent of the benefit plan is to assure me quality care with easy accessibility, which your ruling does not allow. I have found out that there is case law which says that the ERISA exemption is not necessarily final. (See Rebaldo vs. Cuomo, 749 F. 2d 133-1984).* State law does not force the insurance company to allow for additional benefits, only that the insured can choose their provider for an already covered benefit.

Thus, since mental health services are an approved benefit under **(Insurance company name)**, any of the providers named in the Insurance Code must be reimbursed if they are legally qualified to perform the covered services.

---

*Leslie, D., *Insurance Compensation Manual*, 1988.

TABLE 4.1 *(Continued)*

Furthermore, since licensing of health care providers is under state jurisdiction, and I assume that federal law does not currently license such providers, I can only think that Congress did not mean for ERISA to preempt state law regarding mental health providers.

Please reconsider your denial. I appreciate the prompt attention to this matter. I await your reply.
Sincerely,

Client signs and sends

TABLE 4.2   Application Letter to Provider Relations of MCC

LETTERHEAD

Date
Insurance Company Name
Provider Relations
Address

Dear Provider Relations Director:
I am writing to you on behalf of (**Name of Therapist**). As unique and qualified mental health professionals, we are interested in being included on your list of mental health providers.

Since 1983, Psychiatric Mental Health Nurses have been given the authority to receive insurance reimbursement for their services according to California law (Insurance Codes 10176, 10177, 11512.8). In 1992, psychiatric mental health clinical nurse specialists have also been added to the list of "psychotherapists" in the California Evidence Code 1010:8. [For outside California, add your own state's insurance codes and evidence codes here.]

Registered nurses (licensed) with Master's degrees in counseling or psychiatric nursing and two years of experience are allowed to provide mental health services to individuals, couples, and families. These nurses may work in private practice or community settings under the Board of Registered Nursing (scope of practice). These Psychiatric Mental Health Nurses are often referred to as Clinical Nurse Specialists and can be nationally certified as such. They have a unique background that allows them to understand the physical, psychological, pharmacological, and social processes that affect the client and family. They draw upon information and research from a variety of fields including nursing, medicine, sociology, psychology, and marriage/family therapy.

Psychiatric mental health nurses are dedicated to giving comprehensive quality care to clients in order to promote both physical and mental health and well-being using preventative, educative, restorative, and therapeutic techniques.

Because they can provide a wide range of health care services, they are cost-effective while ensuring maximum wellness for the total family system. At a time when we face a crisis in our health care system that includes economic factors and access to quality care, nurses are uniquely prepared to help meet the health needs of our nation.

We believe that your clients have the right to choose the mental health provider that best meets their needs. Placing Master's-prepared nurses on your provider lists provides

TABLE 4.2 *(Continued)*

your subscribers with this opportunity, and also complies with California State laws. You may obtain a master list of certified Psychiatric Clinical Nurse Specialists from the American Nurses Association, the State Board of Registered Nursing, or the State Nurses Association.

We appreciate your willingness to address this important issue and I would be happy to speak to you in more depth, or to your chief executive officer if need be. Please contact me directly for further information at (insert your phone number). The application packets can be addressed to me and mailed to our office.

I look forward to hearing from you at your earliest convenience.

Sincerely,

_____

Name of Therapist and Title

_____

TABLE 4.3   Letter to Insurance to Re-Process Refused Claim

LETTERHEAD

Dear Reviewer:

As you may already know, on January 1, 1983, the Insurance Codes of California were amended (Sections 10176, 10177, and 11512.8), stating that insurance companies that function in California must comply with the laws by reimbursing the services of a psychiatric mental health nurse who has a master's degree and two years supervised experience. Furthermore, psychiatric mental health nurses have also been added in 1992 to the list of "psychotherapists" under the California Evidence Code (1010—Chapter 8). [Add your state's insurance codes in place of California codes.]

I am a Certified Psychiatric Mental Health Clinical Nurse Specialist and meet the requirements for reimbursement. Please remit payment for services rendered.

Thank-you.

_____   _____

Name of Therapist   Date

_____

Since these findings, there have been some additions. Please see Appendix A for a complete listing. My research added the rest of the states, but excluded Alabama, Idaho, Kansas, Kentucky, Louisiana, Minnesota, Ohio, Pennsylvania, and Wyoming. For a listing that includes nurse practitioners, write the American Nurses Association (see Appendix C). It is hoped that they will continue to keep abreast of the changes in each state. For a listing of major insurance companies and managed care companies, their addresses, and contact people, please see Table 4.4. If you have complaints about an insurance company, then you can contact the Insurance Commissioner in your state, by dialing information in the state's capital city. For the California Commissioner contact: Department of Insurance, State of California, 600 South Commonwealth Avenue, Los Angeles, CA 90005, (800) 927-4357 OR 700 L Street, Third Floor, Sacramento, CA 95814.

TYPES OF INSURANCE

There are basically four major types of insurance, not including Medicare, Medicaid (MediCal), Champus, or FEHBP (Federal Employee Health Benefit Plan). These latter ones will be covered later.

I will not discuss Health Maintenance Organizations (HMOs) because they will not reimburse you unless they contract outside of their organization, which is very rare. To become a provider for an HMO, one needs to join the organization and become employed directly by them. Contact the Provider Relations or Human Resources directly for an application. They will not employ you as a private practice clinician. I will discuss Preferred Provider Organizations (PPOs) later in this chapter under the heading "Managed Care." For a copy of the insurance codes, contact the SBRN and/or the Insurance Commissioner in your state. In California, only the indemnity and hospital service contract insurance plans are governed by California's "Freedom of Choice Laws" (see section 10176, 10176.7, 10177, 10177.8, 11512.97, and 11512.8—see end of chapter 1 for complete text). These laws are also printed in the California Board of Registered Nursing handbook under Insurance Codes, or can be found for all the states (if they have them) in most public libraries.[3] Please see Table 4.5 (p. 77–78) for a complete listing of all California laws governing reimbursement.

These California laws came out of Assembly Bills 2211 and 174, and basically say that if an insurance contract offers mental-health coverage to a California resident, then the subscriber has the right/freedom to choose the provider of their choice—psychiatrist, psychologist, licensed clinical social worker, marriage, family and child counselor, and psychiatric mental-health nurses. Nurses were added to this listing in 1982. Furthermore, nurses were given psychotherapist/patient privilege in the California Evidence Code (Section 1010.8) by way of California Assembly Bill 3035 in 1992. Please be sure to read the following section a couple of times because it is essential that you understand which kind of plan your

TABLE 4.4   Insurance/Managed Care Companies

(*Managed Care/PPOs.)
(+Accept nurses in their networks.)
This is only a partial national listing. For a complete state by state national listing, please see, *Psychotherapy Finances: Managed Care Handbook*. Also, check with your own state Insurance Commissioner or Nurses Association for information. The BRNs ususally do not have information on this.

+AETNA
P.O. Box 12340
Fresno, CA 93765

+AETNA HEALTH PLANS
Champus Division/Mental Health Services
16855 W. Bernardo #306
San Diego, CA 92127
(800) 451-8552

*+ALLNET PREFERRED PROVIDER
7777 Center Ave. #490
Huntington Beach, CA 92647
(714) 893-0505

*ALTA HEALTH STRATEGIES INC.
P.O. Box 27317
Salt Lake City, UT 84127
(800) 228-5659

*AMERICAN BIODYNE
400 Oyster Point Blvd. #306
San Francisco, CA 94080
(415) 742-9088

*+AMERICAN PSYCH
MANAGEMENT
Susie Johnson
2400 Broadway Ave.
Santa Monica, CA 90404
(800) 942-4276

*+AMERICAN PSYCH SYSTEMS
6701 Demorary Blvd. #410
Bethseda, MD 20817
(301) 530-4222

*+BEHAVIORAL HEALTH ACCESS
(Blue Cross Managed Care)
P.O. Box 4137
Woodland Hills, CA 9l365

*+BEHAVIORAL HEALTH
RESOURCES
Mary Stokes
P.O. Box 20009
Riverside, CA 92516-009
(800) 451-8552

+BLUE CROSS OF CALIFORNIA
P.O. Box 68006
Anaheim Hills, CALIFORNIA 92817
(800) 451-8552

BLUE CROSS OF WN/ALASKA
P.O. Box 91080
Seattle, WA 98111
(206) 670-4000

BC/BS OF NY (EMPIRE)
P.O. Box 5005
Middletown, NY 10940-9005

+BLUE SHIELD OF CALIFORNIA
Mr. Karl Anderson
Director Allied Health
P.O. Box 7168
San Francisco, CALIFORNIA 94120

+BLUE SHIELD OF CALIFORNIA
P.O. Box 2000
Red Bluff, CA 96080

*CALIFORNIA FOUNDATION FOR
MEDICAL CARE
101 Market St., #610
San Francisco, CALIFORNIA 94105
(415) 957-0618

*CALIFORNIA PREFERRED
PROVIDERS
201 N. Salsipuedes #206
Santa Barbara, CA 93103
(805) 963-0566

TABLE 4.4 (*Continued*)

*CALIFORNIA PSYCH HEALTH
5750 Wilshire Blvd, #490
Los Angeles, CA 90036
(213) 937-9688

CARE-AMERICA
20500 Nordhoff
Chatsworth, CA 90036
(800) 227-3487
(HMO)

CHAMPUS—see Foundation Health Plans

*+CIGNA–CALIFORNIA
2400 East Katella Blvd., Suite 250-A
Anaheim, CA 92806
(714) 939-5600

*+COMMUNITY CARE NETWORK
8911 Balboa Ave.
San Diego, CA 92123

*COMPCARE/HEALTHCARE
750 River Point Drive
West Sacramento, CA 95606
(916) 924-5200

+CONNECTICUT GENERAL
P.O. Box 85455
San Diego, CA 92138

COSTCARE
17011 Beach Blvd.
Huntington Beach, CA 92647

*ETHIX NE
601 Union St. #4330
Seattle, WA 98101
(206) 447-0757

*ETHIX PACIFIC
12655 SW Center St. #180
Beaverton, OR 97005
(503) 641-5352

+FEDERAL EXPRESS
Group Health Adm.
P.O. Box 727
Memphis, TN 38194-9320

*FIRST CHOICE HEALTH PLANS
1100 Olive Wy, #1480
Seattle, WA 98011
(303) 889-3519

*+FOUNDATION HEALTH PLANS
(FHP)
(In the last few months, they have acquired CHAMPUS, Managed Health Network, Health Management Center and Pacific Care.)
Psychcare Services, Inc.
1600 Los Gamos Dr., Suite 300
San Rafael, CA 94903
(415) 491-7200

*GREAT WEST-CARE/LA
8505 E. Orchard Rd.
Englewood, CO 80111
(303) 889-3519

*GREAT WEST-CARE/PORTLAND
8505 E. Orchard Rd.
Englewood, CO 80111
(303) 889-3519

*GREAT WEST-CARE/SEATTLE
8505 E. Orchard Rd.
Englewood, CO 80111
(303) 889-3000

*+HEALTH MANAGEMENT CENTER
Kem Byrn
18000 Studebaker Rd. #690
Cerritos, CA 90701
(800) 327-4103
(see Foundation Health Plans)

*HEALTHNET–
c/o Am. Psy. Management.

*+HELPNET
Julie Escoto
P.O. Box 3217
Long Beach, CA 90803
(800) 435-7638

*HOLMAN GROUP
Cherie Dollins
6900 Owensmouth
Canoga Park, CA 91303
(800) 321-2843

TABLE 4.4 (*Continued*)

+HOME LIFE INS.
P.O. Box 956353
Duluth, GA 30136

*+INTEGRATED BEHAVIORAL
HEALTH
95 Argonaut #200
Laguna Hills, CA 92656
(714) 588-2688

IPSA
Nancy Fagan
1060 San Bernadino Rd.
Upland, CA 91786
(714) 985-1920

+JOHN HANCOCK MUTUAL LIFE
P.O. Box 833859
Richardson, TX 75083-3859

*KINGS COUNTY/BLUE SHIELD
PREFERRED PLAN
1800 Terry Ave.
Seattle, WA 98111
(206) 464-3635

*LIFE-LINK
La Rue Birmingham
23046 Avenida De la Carlotta #700
Laguna Hills, CA 92653
(800) 999-9585

+LINCOLN NATIONAL EMPLOYEES
HEALTH PLAN
Green Bay, WI 54344

*MANAGED CARE NETWORK
700 Pringle Parkway #300
Salem, OR 97302
(503) 371-3249

*MANAGED HEALTHCARE NW
2701 NW Vaughn #710
Portland, OR 97210

*+MANAGED HEALTH NETWORK
(Has merged with Foundation Health as of
June 1, 1996; see above listing)
Dena Chatwin
5100 W. Goldleaf Circle #300
Los Angeles, CA 90056
(800) 777-9355

+MANUFACTURER'S HANOVER
Linwood Group
P.O. Box 9000
Linwood, NJ 08221

*+METLIFE HEALTHCARE
NETWORK
4500 E. Pacific Coast Hwy. #600
Long Beach, CA 90804
(310) 597-9932

++METRAHEALTH
(Has joined with Traveler's and Metropoli-
tan Life; later this year will join with United
HealthCare Corp. (UHC) and United Be-
havioral Systems (UBS)).
P.O. Box 22026
Albany, NY 12201-2026
(518) 454-4500

+METROPOLITAN LIFE
Chris Ciano
4500 Pacific Coast hwy. #120
Long Beach, CA 90804-3271

*+MUTUAL OF OMAHA MUTUALLY
PREFERRED
10 Universal City Plaza #1920
Universal City, CA 91608

+NORTHWESTERN NATIONAL LIFE
730 Fairmont Ave. #202
Glendale, CA 91203

*+OCCUPATIONAL HEALTH SERV.
Vickie Ina
125 E. Sir Francis Drake Blvd. #300
Larkspur, CA 94939-1860

+OPERATING ENGINEER'S
HEALTH & WELFARE FUND
P. O. Box 7067
Pasadena, CA 91109
(818) 356-1004

*+OUCH
5777 W. Century Blvd., #1500
Los Angeles, CA 90045

+PARTNER'S
P.O. Box 50031
San Bernadino, CA 92412
(800) 541-7832

(Continued)

TABLE 4.4 (*Continued*)

*PACC PREFERRED
12901 SE 97TH Ave.
Clackamas, OR 97015
(503) 659-4212

*+PERS-CARE/BLUE SHEILD PPO
P.O. Box 92945
Los Angeles, CA 90009-2945
(310) 670-8870

*+PREFERRED HEALTH CARE
Susan Reimer/Phil Sorley
P.O. Box 19553
Irvine, CA 92713
(800) 228-1286

*PREFERRED HEALTH NETWORK
301 E. Ocean Blvd. #900
Long Beach, CA 90802
(310) 983-1616

*PM GROUP/PACIFIC MUTUAL
700 Newport Center Dr.
Newport Beach, CA 92660
(714) 760-4383

*PREFERRED PROVIDER PLAN
BLUE CROSS/BLUE SHIELD
P.O. Box 1271
Portland, OR 97207
(503) 225-5280

PRINCIPAL MUTUAL
5030 Camino de la Siesta #301
San Diego, CA 92108

+PRUDENTIAL
P.O. Box 500
Mt. Arlington, NJ 07856

+*PRUNET/PRUDENTIAL
P.O. Box 500
Mt. Arlington, NJ 07856

*PSYCHADVANTAGE INC.
6377 Riverside Ave., #170
Riverside, CA 92506

*+SANA Psychological & Health, Inc.
Ms. Ellen Jones
1355 Westwood Blvd., #10
Los Angeles, CA 90024

*SAN JOAQUIN FOUNDATION
P.O. Box 21002
Stockton, CA 95210
(209) 951-4560

*TAKECARE HEALTH PLAN
21700 Oxnard St. #2500
Woodland Hills, CA 9l367
(818) 716-7033
(HMO)

+TRAVELER'S INS.
1 Point Drive #600
Brea, CA 92621
(800) 243-0191

+TRAVELER'S PPO
*Uses US Behavioral Health
(800) 255-6053

+UNITED INSURANCE COMPANY OF
AMERICA
P.O. Box 4270
Woodland Hills, CA 91365-4270

*UNITED NW SERVICES
P.O. Box 141253
Spokane, WA 99214
(509) 928-2569

+UNITED OF OMAHA
P.O. Box 1332
Spokane, WA 99214

*+USA HEALTHNET
7301 N. 16th St. #210
Phoenix, AZ 85020

*+U.S. BEHAVIORAL HEALTH (USBH)
425 Market St., 27th Floor
San Francisco, CA 94105
(800) 333-8724

VICTIM'S WITNESS
STATE BOARD OF CONTROL
P.O. Box 48
Sacramento, CA 95812

*+VALUE BEHAVIORAL HEALTH
P.O. Box 7203
Wilton, CT 06897–7203
(800) 435–3231

client has so that you get reimbursed in a timely manner. Even though your state may have different insurance codes or none at all, these definitions for types of insurance will apply nationally. Many states have a type or form of "Freedom of Choice Laws," which disallow for any particular type of provider to be discriminated against. It is beyond the scope of this book to address each individual state's insurance codes; California is offered as an example only. Please see Appendix A for individual state reimbursement information.

TABLE 4.5 California PMHNs Right to Practice and Reimbursement by Third-Party Payors

---

The Insurance Commission has jurisdiction over all insurance companies which operate in the state of California, based on the Insurance Code of California.[4] The Corporation Commission has jurisdiction over all managed care corporations, as defined by the *Knox-Keene* Health Care Service Plan Act of 1975, based on the Health and Safety Code.[5] These are the only two sets of law that govern health care. Any company must abide by one set of laws or the other. Furthermore, the laws were written to be complementary. Within the Health and Safety Code is this provision:

1342.5 Consultation with Insurance Commissioner. The commissioner shall consult with the Insurance Commissioner prior to adopting any regulations applicable to health care service plans . . . for the specific purpose of ensuring, to the extent practical, that there is consistency of regulations applicable to these plans and entities by the Insurance Commissioner and the Commissioner of Corporations.

Insurance Codes

10176 Medical reimbursement provisions of disability policies. In disability insurance, the policy may provide for payment of mental health expenses. No such policy shall prohibit the insured from selecting any registered nurse licensed pursuant to Chapter 6 (commencing with Section 2700) of Division 2 of the Business and Professions Code who possesses a master's degree in psychiatric mental-health nursing and two years of supervised experience in psychiatric mental-health nursing.

10177 Mental health coverage in self-insured employee welfare benefit plan. No such plan shall prohibit the employee from selecting any registered nurse licensed pursuant to Chapter 6 (commencing with Section 2700) of Division 2 of the Business and Professions Code who possesses a master's degree in psychiatric mental-health nursing and two years of supervised expeience in psychiatric mental-health nursing.

11512.8 Professional mental health coverage. A hospital service contract may provide for payment of professional mental health expenses of any registered nurse licensed pursuant to Chapter 6 (commencing with Section 2700) of Division 2 of the Business and Professions Code who possesses a master's degree in psychiatric-mental health nursing and two years of supervised experience in psychiatric-mental health nursing.

TABLE 4.5 *(Continued)*

10133.6. This section does not change existing *antitrust law* as it relates to any agreement or arrangement to exclude from any of the above-descirbed groups or combinations any person who is lawfully qualified to perform the services to be performed by the members of the group or combination where the ground for the exclusion is *failure to possess the same license* or certification as is possessed by the members of the group or combination.

10180. Duty to give reasonable consideration to proposals for contracting. (a) A disability insurer which negotiates and enters into a contract with professional providers . . . shall give reasonable consideration to timely written proposals for contracting by licensed or certified professional providers. ''Reasonable consideration'' means consideration in good faith . . . proposal for contracting prior to the time that contracts are entered into or renewed. An insurer may specify the terms and conditions of contracting to assure cost efficiency, qualification of providers, appropriate utilization of services, accessibility, convenience to persons who would receive the provider's services, and consistency with its basic method of opeation, but *shall not exclude providers because of their category of license.*

Health and Safety Codes

1373[h][iii]. No plan shall prohibit the member from selecting any registered nurse licensed pursuant to Chapter 6 (commencing with Section 2700) of Division 2 of the Business and Professions code who possesses a master's degree in psychiatric mental-health nursing and two years of supervised experience in psychiatric mental-health nursing.

1373.8 Contractees' right to select licensed professionals in California to perform contract services. A health care service plan contract which includes California residents but which may be written or issued for delivery outside of California, where benefits are provided within the scope of practice of a registered nurse licensed pursuant to chapter 6 (commencing with Section 2700) of Division 2 of the Business and Professions Code who possesses a master's degree in psychiatric mental-health nursing and two years of supervised experience in psychiatric mental-health nursing . . . shall not be deemed to prohibit persons covered under the contract from selecting those licensed persons in California.

1342.6 Effect of antitrust prohibitions on health care services. This section does not change existing *antitrust law* as it relates to any agreement or arrangement to exclude from any of the above-described groups or combinations any person who is lawfully qualified to perform the services to be performed by the members of the group or combination where the ground for the exclusion is *failure to possess the same license* or certification as is possessed by the members of the group or combination.

1373.9 Duty to give reasonable consideration to proposals for affiliation. (a) A health care service plan which negotiates and enters into a contract with professional providers . . . shall give reasonable consideration to timely written proposals for affiliation by licensed or certified professional providers. ''Reasonable consideration'' means consideration in good faith . . . proposals for affiliation prior to the time that contracts are entered into or renewed. A plan may specify the terms and conditions of affiliation to assure cost efficiency, qualifications of providers, appropriate utilization of services, accessibility, convenience to persons who would receive the provider's services, and consistency with the plan's basic method of operation, but *shall not exclude providers because of their category of license.*

Indemnity Benefit Plans

These are the most common and are also referred to as Disability Health and Life plans and are designed to reimburse subscribers directly for expenses incurred. Some examples of major indemnity plans are Aetna, Traveler's, and Prudential. These all fall within the definition of an insurance company and are therefore bound by state laws, even if the company is based outside of the home state. (See 10176 and 10176.7 of the California Insurance Code for example.)

It has been my experience that these companies are sometimes the easiest to get reimbursement from for nurses. I have been reimbursed by the following Indemnity Benefit plans: Aetna, John Hancock, Mutual of Omaha, Northwest National Life, Metropolitan Life, Connecticut General, United Insurance Company of America, Principal Mutual, and National Health Service, to name a few. Although these have been relatively open to reimbursing nurses, by and large, they are going to managed care companies for cost-effectiveness and this often makes it harder to get reimbursement (see section on managed care).

Health Care Service Plans

These are prepaid health plans and work very much like the Indemnity plans. The major one that you should be concerned about is Blue Shield. Currently, Blue Shield of California does recognize and reimburse the services of psychiatric mental-health nurses, but they will not reimburse directly. Instead, they will send the payment to the client and you will have to collect from them. I have been told by the director of Blue Shield that this is changing. I honestly don't think it will change in the next few years until the number of PMHNs is significant.

Please remember that these plans are more particular about having a physician's referral (see billing information). These plans as well as managed care companies are regulated by the Department of Corporations, so they are not obliged to follow state laws, though this may be changing over the next few years. For complaints, contact this department (see address under managed care).

Therefore, Blue Shield from other states does not have to acknowledge you as a provider. Still, it doesn't hurt to write to them to clarify your right to practice and to attempt reimbursement, especially if they utilize other master's-prepared clinicians, such as marriage, family and child counselors, or social workers.

I have been reimbursed by Blue Shield of California through my clients, including their Preferred Provider Organization (PPO), Pers-Care. As of yet, PMHNs are not considered participating providers and so reimbursement will be sent directly to the client, not the provider. This is the policy of Blue Shield. Hopefully, PMHNs will soon be considered fully. You must remember to apply first for a Blue Shield provider number to ensure ease of reimbursement. Your billing should always include this number. This is separate from becoming part of their PPO, and does not mean you are considered a participating provider. The California address is: Blue Shield of California, Provider Relations, P.O. Box 797, Turlock, CA 95381-0797.

Hospital Service Plans

For the most part, these will be Blue Cross plans. I have not had any trouble being reimbursed by Blue Cross of California, including the PPO (Behavioral Health Access/BHA). These plans fall under California state law and the Department of Insurance also (see Insurance Code 11512.3, 11512.8). These plans work essentially the same as indemnity plans.

You just need to be careful, as with all of the insurance companies, that you are working directly with them or if you have a PPO/managed care company taking over for them. Be sure to understand this so that you can explain the relevance of the insurance codes to the out-of-state Blue Cross plan as well (see above codes).

Self-Insured Welfare Benefit Plans

This is the last major type of insurance. It is by far the hardest from which to get reimbursement. They are services directly provided by the employer or through a union. Sometimes they are administrated by another insurance company; for example: Hertz, Operating Engineers Trust Fund, and Commercial Works Union. These plans fall under the jurisdiction of ERISA (Employee Retirement Income Security Act of 1975). I have a friend who has been paid by the Federal Express (SIWP), and I am working with Hertz on a rejected claim at present.

This means that they are for the most part unaffected by the state laws, although there has been some case law that seems to point out that they really are not exempt if they cover mental health services under their plans.[6] They do not have to offer mental-health services by law, as do the regular insurance companies. If they do, you may have a case to argue for your reimbursement, especially if they cover other master's-prepared clinicians (see Table 4.5).

If they do not limit the provider, that is, they include an MD- or PhD-level provider only, then you have a stronger case and should protest. Just be careful to realize that whatever they say probably will hold. Your client can take them to court if they so choose, but I wouldn't recommend it. There are some encouraging signs that there is a strong movement for having more controls over managed care and the self-insured plans to make them more accountable to state laws. Until then, however, it is imperative that YOU call the insurance company prior to seeing the client, or at least as soon after as possible to check on benefits before you incur any expenses. This is particularly true in cases where the person has managed care and you see the client before calling the plan. In this case, they won't authorize or pay for services. Most people don't know whether they have an HMO, PPO, or regular indemnity insurance.

Taking the initiative will greatly reduce time wasted and future headaches when you are denied a claim. It is difficult and unpleasant to end therapy with a client after many sessions because their insurance won't pay. It is your ethical responsibility as patient advocate to help the client to understand and gain access to their coverage, but it is also a matter of self-preservation! Furthermore, be sure to have the client sign a release of information and assignment of benefits (AOB) to you on one of their claim forms or on a master that you have created. This form must be sent in with the first billing (see Billing, page 87).

Finally, don't be afraid to bill anyway, just in case they do pay. Insurance companies are not always consistent or logical. Don't be afraid to call and talk to the provider relations department, or to send them information about nurses or copies of the laws. For first time billing, it may be helpful to send a copy of the Fact Sheet (Table 2.1), brochure, and business card.

OTHER TYPES OF HEALTH COVERAGE

Medicare

I will only discuss Medicare briefly, and only as it relates to outpatient mental health services. Medicare is regulated by federal law under the Health Care Financing Administration (HCFA), and so is exempt from the state laws (although each state is responsible for administering of the funds).

Medicare is basically health coverage for those over 65 years of age, or those who are chronically disabled (including chronically mentally ill). It consists of Part A (hospital expenses) and Part B (out-patient services). In January of 1991, clinical nurse specialists were recognized providers of services, and new federal regulations provided for reimbursement of all services. Currently, they will directly reimburse independent nurse practitioners and clinical nurse specialists in skilled nursing facilities and other settings *in federally designated rural areas only* (non-Metropolitan). Certified nurse midwives and registered nurse anesthetists are also covered. They will reimburse for all services in nonrural areas only with "Incident to" provisions, meaning that the nurse must be employed by a physician, who bills directly to Medicare under his or her Medicare number. Please call your local HCFA for a listing of designated rural locations in your state.

Generally, the federal regulations do acknowledge advanced practice nurses, but they do say that it is up to each individual state to specify the definition of clinical nurse specialists. Currently, the California Board of Registered Nursing has not done so. Therefore, only rural CNSs and NPs can bill independently at present, unless "Incident to" another provider (see Incident to).

Billing must be done on a standard HCFA 1500 form, and you must first obtain a Medicare provider number. The California Nurses Association is encouraging all advanced practice nurses to apply for a number so that when the legislation is passed, they will be able to bill. The number for California is: MediCare Provider Certification, P.O. Box 797, Turlock, CA 05381-0797; or call (213) 742-3843, 742-3945 (Southern CA); (209) 634-9119 (all others).

The MediCare carriers for California are: MediCare Transamerica, Occidental Insurance Co., P. O. Box 50061, Upland, CA 91785-5061, (800) 675-2266, (213) 748-2311 (counties of L. A., Orange, San Diego, Imperial).

For the rest of the state: MediCare Claims Department, Blue Shield of California, Chico, CA 95976, (800) 848-7713.

Medicare will generally pay 75% to 85% of physician fees for advanced practice nursing services.[7] This last year failed to pass a new law that would increase Medicare funds to 97% of physician fees. It is hoped that Senate Bills 2103, and 2104, and House of Representatives Bills 4962 and 4963 will be reintroduced and passed with this Clinton administration. As of yet, it has not gone through.

Furthermore, in 1994, HCFA mandated that Nurse Practitioners and Clinical Nurse Specialists have UPINS (Unique Provider Identification Numbers). These have always been required of physicians, and it is the HCFA's way of tracking fraud and abuse cases across state lines. Until you get one, you need to use the digits "oth000" on the form.[8]

The other mechanism by which advanced practice nurses can receive reimbursement by Medicare–Part B is through the "Incident To" provision. This means that you can be paid for your services if you are working with a physician, psychologist, or social worker who is an approved Medicare provider (i.e., has a provider number).

There are certain criteria, though, that must be met. First, you must be employed by the provider directly or by a joint agency. That person must serve in a supervisory capacity and be on-site while giving services, but they don't have to be in the same room. He or she must be available to provide assistance if need be, however.[9] There also must be a formal written relationship between the parties.

These services are billed under the physician's or other practitioner's UPIN and Medicare number, although there is a place on the form to designate that the services were performed by a nonphysician practitioner (although most don't put this on the form and Medicare says that they don't want the name of the employee on the form). I think it is important so that advanced practice nurse services can be traced and researched. How else will we be able to show quality and cost effectiveness?

It is important that whoever performs the services should be identified, even if there is a supervisory relationship (see Billing on following pages). There should be a place on your master bill to show who performed the service, and who is the supervisor, if applicable. Not clearly divulging this information may be interpreted as insurance fraud. This is particularly the case when the insurance plan does not cover your services. You can't submit a bill under someone else's license/name even if they are the supervisor. This is fraud when done with regular insurance claims, and has been a prosecutable issue,[10] but Medicare seems to encourage this practice. If you are billing "Incident to," it is wise to contact your local carrier for written guidelines. You can also obtain guidelines for billing from HCFA. Sometimes, a carrier may tell you to bill under the Current Procedural Terminology code 99211 when the service is provided by a "nonphysician."[11] The problem with this is that it is intended for a brief five-minute intervention and really doesn't cover most services. It is best to use the CPT code that appropriately reflects the level of care provided, regardless of the type of provider (see Billing on following pages).

Medicaid

Medicaid (MediCal in California) is regulated by federal law–Title 19 of the Social Security Act under the Health Care Financing Administration (HCFA). It then is interpreted and carried out by state regulatory agencies and laws. It basically provides health care for the poor and needy.

As with Medicare, advanced practice nurses have been slow to be recognized as valid providers. Oregon, Washington, and Arizona have legislation that provides for Family and Pediatric Nurse Practitioners.[12] Please see your individual state section for specifics.

In 1994, California Assembly Bill 1224 passed, which qualified direct reimbursement to Family and Pediatric Nurse Practitioners. Certified nurse midwives are also covered in California. Currently, clinical nurse specialists are not specifically named for direct reimbursement except in Florida, Minnesota, Texas, and Wisconsin (although there was a bill up for Congress in 1993 which failed). On July 1, 1994 the Senate Finance Committee voted to provide outpatient Medicare reimbursement for all nurse practitioners regardless of geographical area.[13] This bill was to include direct reimbursement to CNSs as well, but was eliminated to keep costs low. This legislation would override the state's practice acts and offer a tax credit for those NPs who practice in underserved areas. For a listing of state by state Medicaid reimbursement write the American Nurses Association, Division of Governmental Affairs, 600 Maryland Avenue, Suite 100 West, Washington, DC 20024-2571, (202) 554-4444. You may write or call the following for information about working under another MediCal provider (request Form MC 1201). For an application for a MediCal provider number, you can ask for Form MC4032. Department of Health Services, Provider Enrollment Services, 714 P St. Room 940, P.O. Box 942732, Sacramento, CA 94234-7320, (916) 323-1945. It would behoove you to stay abreast of current federal and state laws that would affect nursing practice. *Nurseweek*, the *California Nurse*, the *American Nurse*, and especially *Capitol Update* can all be good resources (see Appendix B, page 142).

Champus

Champus stands for Civilian Health and Medical Program of the Uniformed Services and covers the military and their dependents. Currently, Champus is underwritten in California by Foundation Health Plans. Champus acknowledges the services of nurse practitioners, nurse midwives, registered nurse anesthetists, and clinical nurse specialists (psychiatric mental health only.) Certified psychiatric nurse specialists can provide services independent of a physician referral and supervision, but it is useful to continue to get the referral in writing just in case. You must get a Champus provider number no matter what. They also are moving to a form of managed care that requires authorization for more than two sessions a week and treatment of more than 23 sessions a year. Claims may be filed as follows:

Foundation Health Plans/Champus; Psychcare Services, 1600 Los Gamos Dr., Suite 300, San Rafael, CA 94903, (415) 491-7200.

Oregon/Washington, BC/BSSC, P.O. Box 1005202, Florence, SC 29501-0502, (800) 476-8500.

Be sure to call before you send in a claim because the carriers are often changing: Blue Cross of Washington/Alaska used to handle California claims, so you must keep current. Call your local Champus to find out specifics for your state. When billing, please use the white Champus form 501/HCFA 1500.

There are some changes involving mental health services and a new Army managed care program is called "Gateway to Care" which will include some preventative services, day treatment, weekend services, and so forth. There is also another managed care program called Champus Select (a special PPO). For information on the new rules and the managed care programs as they relate to mental health, you can contact:

CHAMP-MH, P.O. Box 26307, Alexandria, VA 22313, (800) 242-6764.

Currently, Aetna/Champus for California is not taking any new providers for their Champus Prime program, but they frequently assess a need for new providers.

FEHBP

FEHBP stands for Federal Employee Health Benefit Plan and is open to all employees of the government. There are two types of plans. One is a services benefit plan through Blue Cross or Blue Shield (in California). The other is an indemnity benefit plan, that is, a commercial insurance plan (see indemnity plans, p. 79). You should check with the client's specific plan to assess which type of coverage is offered.

Public law 101-509, which allows direct reimbursement to nurse mid-wives, nurse practitioners, registered nurse anesthetists, and clinical nurse specialists without supervision or referral, was passed in 1990.[14] Where the client seeks help outside of an HMO, there must be a doctor's referral. I have billed FEHBP through Blue Shield of California with success. When billing, use a master bill and an insurance claims form from the carrier, which the client should provide.

California Victims of Crime

If you practice in California at this time, it is important for you to know that Victims of Crime via the State Board of Control will not reimburse Psychiatric Mental Health Nurses. They will directly reimburse marriage, family and child counselors and licensed clinical social workers. The California Nurses Association has called for a ruling about this position as it relates to psychiatric mental-health nurses by the Office of Administrative Law.[15] Check your own state government for a Victims of Crime program. The following relates to the California program only. In the past, they have reimbursed nurses who have had the bills co-signed by another supervising licensed provider (not another nurse). They now say that they will not reimburse nurses even with this countersignature. The reasons they have stated are that the California laws specifically mandate who they can reimburse, and nurses are not now currently listed. So, be wary in taking on Victim Witness clients, although we as nurses are uniquely qualified to treat them (especially sexual assault victims). If you do work with them be aware of the following. Make sure your clients fill out an application as soon as possible with the local Victim Witness program or have them do one through you. It takes about five weeks after receiving the application before the client will have a number assigned to them at VW. Furthermore, do not send any bills to them until after they have given your client a number. Call them in Sacramento or call the local Victim Witness Program through the district attorney's (D.A.) office to find out the number after it has been placed in the computer. You can contact them for information, applications, and VW Billing forms at:

State Board of Control, Victims of Crime Program, P. O. Box 3036, Sacramento, CA 95812-3036, (800) 777-9229. Call your local district attorney's office for information.

Then, you may submit bills. Be sure to use the green forms along with your master bill. The client must sign the green forms. If the submitted form is not signed, they will send your bills back to you and thus further delay your payments.

As it stands now, it will take between six months or a year to actually receive any payments. It will probably take about six months just to hear back from them that they are processing the claims. They are having severe financial difficulty and so payments may be delayed as long as 18 months.

Remember, a victim has only one year from the date of the crime to file an application. There can be some exceptions to this if the victim is a minor. My experience has been that if they can find a reason to deny your claim, they will. So be careful.

Also, be aware that in September 1992, the laws were passed that say if you accept VW funds for payment, you cannot try to collect the difference from your clients between what VW pays and your usual and customary bill. For example, if your fees are $100 per session and VW now pays $70 per session, you cannot bill the client for the $30.00 difference. Be clear with your client as to what you will do if VW does not pay, and that they may have accumulated a bill that could possibly be in the thousands by the time that you hear about the denial. Remember, you can't write off bad debts or unpaid bills on your taxes.

Some people refuse to bill the client, others pursue it. You may count this as "pro bono" work. In any case, just be sure to inform your client fully. It has been my experience that the local Project Sister (Sexual Assault Center) in our area tends to be overly confident about reimbursement. Finally, there is now a 50-session limit for postvictimization counseling.

BILLING

In order to get reimbursed for your services in a timely manner, you need to be aware of some important aspects of billing. First, you need a billing form (see Tables 4.6 and 4.7). You can make your own, adapt the one in this book, or buy a computer program. I use LotusWorks for mine and it is incredibly quick and looks professional.

The following is essential information that a bill should contain:

PROVIDER INFORMATION
Agency/provider name
SS# or Tax or Employer Identity Number (TIN/EIN)
Billing and place of service address

Provider phone number

Provider license type, credentials, and certification numbers (Include special provider numbers, i.e., Blue Shield)

Assignment of benefits (Provider—Signature on File) or Client

Place of service (0 = office, 1 = hospital)

Service Rendered—Current Procedural Codes (see CPT, p. 94)

Dates of Service

Cost of service, amount client paid, and balance due

Date bill prepared (must be after the last billed session)

Who performed therapy

Your signature and supervisor if applies

CLIENT INFORMATION

Name of insured

Name of client and relationship to above

Address

SS# of insured

Employer/Insurance company name

Group/Employee/identification number

Referral source where applicable (doctor)

Date of birth

Diagnosis (use DSM IV–Axis I & II)

Be sure to attach a filled out insurance claim form or Assignment of Benefits/Release of Information Form (Table 4.8) the first time that you submit a bill. After that, you can just indicate "Signature on file," so the insurance company will reimburse you instead of the client. They sometimes send the money to the client anyway, so be sure to collect from them and remind them of this.

Absolutely remember to attach a *copy* (not the original) of any managed care authorization forms for the dates of services each time you bill. They will not pay for anything unless they have this in hand. Sometimes this gets lost, so be sure to keep the original. It really can prolong your payment if you don't do this.

TABLE 4.6   Manual Insurance Billing Form

Insured_____ Name of Client_____

Insured SS#_____

Client DOB_____Employer_____

Place of Service_____

Date first seen for this condition_____

Has patient ever had same or similiar condition?_____

Diagnosis: Axis I_____

_____

          Axis II_____

_____90844 Ind. Therapy _____99221 Initial OP Eval.

_____90846 Conjoint Therapy _____99222 Inpt. TX.

_____90847 Family Therapy _____99223 Inpt. TX.

_____90857 Group Therapy _____99361 Team Conferences

_____90889 Special Reports _____90830 Psychological Testing

Total # of Sessions: _____Total Fees_____
Date(s) of Treatment for Month of _____19_____

1 2 3 4 5 6 7 8 9 10 11 12 13 14 15 16 17 18 19 20 21 22 23 24 25 26 27 28 29 30 31
Name of Agency

Address

Phone Number

Employer ID# (if applies)

_____Name of Therapist   _____Name of Therapist

     License Numbers   License Numbers

     SS#   SS#

Provider's Signature _____

Supervisor's Signature _____

TABLE 4.7   Sample Billing Form

PLACE OF SERVICE:
ADDRESS OF SERVICE PROVIDER
CITY, STATE, ZIP CODE
PHONE NUMBER

STATEMENT OF SERVICES

Insured:	Insured ID No:
Address:	Patient:
	Date of Birth: / /
Employer/Ins:	Group No:
Referral Source:	Employee No:

Diagnostic   Axis I:
Impression:
                 Axis II:

Date of Service	Place	Service Rendered	Charge:
/ /	0	Individual Therapy (90844)	
/ /	0	Individual Therapy (90844)	
//	0	Individual Therapy (90844)	
/ /	0	Individual Therapy (90844)	
/ /	0	Individual Therapy (90844)	
			Total:

Past Due:
Amount Paid:
Balance Due:

Date Prepared: / /
Pay Benefits To:

SERVICES PERFORMED BY:

Jane Doe, M.A., R.N., C.S.
Psychiatric Mental-Health
Clinical Nurse Specialist
License #:   CNS#
SS#:   PHN# or PMHN#

TABLE 4.8 Assignment of Benefits/Release of Information Form

LETTERHEAD

AUTHORIZATION/RELEASE OF INFORMATION:

I hereby authorize (insurance company) _____
or its representatives to inspect or secure copies of case history records, diagnosis, prognosis, and any other data covering this claim.

Insured   Date

AUTHORIZATION/ASSIGNMENT OF BENEFITS:

I hereby authorize (insurance company) _____
or its representatives to pay bills in connection with this claim and to remit directly to the Provider as named below for services rendered:

AGENCY NAME
ADDRESS
THERAPIST NAME

Insured   Date

---

of this, and if you are having particular difficulty, then complain to the Insurance Commissioner (see address below). Unfortunately, it can take many months to get your first payment. After you are in their computer as a vendor, subsequent claims are usualy paid within three weeks, sometimes sooner. Remember to be patient and nice to the insurance claims adjusters at all times and to present yourself as a professional. Remain firm; you have the right to practice and to get paid for your services.

Billing really isn't that hard after you get into the system, and you have a billing program. It will become easier as time goes on. By and large, if out-patient therapy is covered, you should get paid (see above types of insurance again). If you haven't received payment within 30 days, then call them to check on the status of your claim. The future trend is toward electronic claim processing and doing away with paper claims. (See section under Billing Tips.)

Always chart when and who you called, and keep the numbers and extensions on your statement form for ease. Try to always use the 800 numbers to keep costs down. Try to work with the same person if you can. The voice-mail system is usually frustrating, and you can spend hours following up on the phone. Try to set aside 30 minutes to an hour every one to two weeks to follow up and make all your calls at once. This will cut down on your frustration level.

Remember, if you bill insurance companies for your client, it's a convenience for them. It is not mandatory, and it is time consuming. You are spending extra time and therefore need to be compensated as such. Some people charge from $5.00 to $20.00 each time insurance is billed. Remember, too, you may not see your money for months. I explain that I am doing this as a courtesy to them, and it is complicated, and deserves compensation. This is one reason to charge your regular fees.

Of course, the ideal is to have your clients pay the full fee, and you bill the insurance company so that the client gets reimbursed. This will save a lot of hours, and gets you the money up front. The problem is that most people can't afford to pay all up front. It is your decision. I suggest that you do this as you can, but not billing insurance companies will hinder your practice. If you work with managed care companies, then you must be prepared to bill.

DIAGNOSIS

Billing insurance companies always requires that the patient have a formal diagnosis (medical, not nursing) written on the billing form. Because some states state that nurses are not allowed to "diagnose," you may write your "diagnostic impression" on the bill. Or, you may use the diagnosis that the patient's physician has used provided they have seen a doctor already. Currently, the system is run on the DSM-IV (*Diagnostic and Statistical Manual*, 4th ed.).[16] If you are not familiar with this text, then you will not be able to bill insurance companies. They only accept diagnoses from this system. Please note that the latest edition came out in May of 1994, and most insurance companies and clinicians will still be using the DSM-III-R version in 1995 and probably later. Do feel free to use either one at this point. It is suggested that you start using the new edition as soon as you feel comfortable with it. It is also helpful to have a little pocket manual at your desk or computer.[17] It makes it easy to use. Make sure that you include both Axis 1 and 2. You often need to add Axis 3–5 to the treatment plans when working with managed care companies that require them. I often use V71.09 (No Diagnosis on Axis II) if the individual does not qualify for a personality disorder. Take a class on pathology or use of the DSM-IV if you didn't get this in your master's program or are weak in this area. Be sure to have a few good texts on hand as references too.[18] Since the new edition came out, many seminars and guides will be available to help you in this area.

Some people are uncomfortable about the use of diagnosis. *Actually, you are not diagnosing.* Only physicians can legally diagnose illness in most states, unless the Nurse Practice Act states that you can specifically diagnose. Many do so for NP's scope of practice. All nurses, even at the basic level are trained in recognition of illness. All nurses formulate a medical diagnosis as well as a nursing diagnosis in assessing and treating patients, but legally it is not considered "diagnosing" unless you have legal jurisdiction to do so in your state. It is one of the aspects of advanced practice that legislation has lagged behind. It shouldn't be a problem unless your state precludes you from third-party billing.

Otherwise, it must be posted on the bill if you want to be reimbursed. All mental-health professionals use this system. You may add your nursing diagnosis if you like, but the insurance companies will not pay for them (at least at present). A very complete guide to nursing diagnosis is Carpenito's *Nursing Diagnosis.*[19] Another good psychiatric text which includes nursing diagnosis plus DSM-III-R is Aromando's *Mental Health and Psychiatric Nursing.*[20]

Another important point is to discuss the diagnosis with the client prior to billing. Clients have the right to know, especially since it becomes a part of their permanent record to pass from insurance company to company. You never know what will become of this information. They must sign a release of information before you bill (to maintain the confidentiality).

I limit the information that I give insurance companies to the least possible. I also try to give the client the least pathological diagnosis possible, that is, Adjustment Disorder with Anxious Mood compared to General Anxiety Disorder. But, it is important to be truthful.

Most insurance companies look at adjustment disorders as benign and situational, so these are what I use a lot, if they are applicable. However, beware that managed care companies are less inclined to give you very many sessions for an adjustment disorder rather than a major disorder.

The process will become easier for you after a few trial runs. Most of the time you won't be asked to provide any more information, except with the managed care companies. They usually want a treatment plan, goals, and strategies. These can be very time-consuming and difficult to put together. Try to be brief and succinct; they prefer behavioral/short-term interventions. Try to be professional and practice filling these out if possible.

Remember also that you should charge every time the insurance company requests further patient information beyond what is on the billing form or simply fill in the blanks type of information. The insurance company will usually pay $25 to $100 for detailed reports and assessment or treatment plans (use CPT code 90889—Treatment Reports).

CPT CODES

This refers to the Current Procedural Terminology which is written for physician services and is commonly used by all mental health professionals. Again, this is an essential part of billing. They are the procedural codes that determine reimbursement by the insurance companies. Like diagnosis, you cannot receive payment for services without use of these. The old California standard nomenclature is outdated and should not be used.

You can get a copy of the latest CPT codes for about $35.00 from: American Medical Association, Book and Pamphlet #0p054190, P.O. Box 10946, Chicago, IL 60610. There are hundreds of codes listed. Here are the ones that you will most frequently use in your counseling practice. Please consult the CPT Code manual for complete descriptions. The codes indicated by an asterisk (*) are most frequently used in billing.

Out-Patient

90801	Psychiatric diagnostic interview and assessment includes history, mental status exam. Please use this for the first time sessions; insurance will usually pay more for this service.
*90844	About 45–50 minutes of individual therapy
*90846	Family therapy without the client present
*90847	Family or marital therapy with the client present
90857	Group therapy
90880	Hypnotherapy
90900	Biofeedback
99050	After hours services
99078	Educational services to groups
90889	Special Reports

90830   Psychological Testing

Please note that some insurance companies will not pay for "couple/marriage/relationship counseling (90847). Please check first with them before seeing the clients. Another option is to bill for individual therapy with one of the partners (90844) even though a spouse or significant other is in the room. Remember that the individual who gets billed will need an individual diagnosis. You can add "Marital Problem" (V61.10) under Axis II Diagnosis. This is perfectly legal.

In-Patient

The most common usage is 90844 and is designated for hospital place of service. Otherwise you may use the following. The numbers in parentheses refer to time in minutes spent with patient.

99221   Initial evaluation and history

99222   Hospital care, per day, moderate complexity

99223   Hospital care, per day, high complexity

99231   Subsequent hospital care, low complexity (15)

99232   Subsequent hospital care, moderate complexity (25)

88233   Subsequent hospital care, per day, high complexity (35)

*99361   Team Conferences

Please see CPT Manual for detailed explanations.

MANAGED CARE

Managed Care is the buzzword for the 1990s, as far as health care goes. With the incredibly escalating costs of health care, insurance companies are turning over their mental health services to managed care companies daily.

Managed care companies are businesses and are therefore subject to the Department of Corporations laws (see Table 4.5). They really don't have to adhere strictly to the state insurance codes because of this. Most though, do try to adhere to the insurance codes in setting up their preferred provider organizations (PPOs).

As mentioned earlier, when a client has health care through a Health Maintenance Organization (HMO), you usually will not be able to bill them for services. The exception may be a temporary authorization of your services when the client is out of their network area. For this, please call the Provider Relations of the HMO. The client's primary care physician must refer to you in this case. Otherwise, the client needs to either pay you out of pocket, or go to their HMO directly for services. For information on how you can become part of a managed care network, please see page 98.

The Way It Works

The essential elements of managed care are that insurance companies need to find a way to limit the services/expenditures of their subscribers by literally managing their case, which is why managed care is so big. The client is assigned a case manager who determines if services are indeed necessary and then refers the client to one of the providers within the network that is within the local geographical area of the client.

Usually Mental Health services can only be acquired by first calling the Managed Care company (MCC) and requesting services.

If You're Not In The Network

Some MCCs will let the client see you even if you are not part of their network, but it can be at a reduced fee. Make sure you check to see if the client has an out-of-network provision. It differs from plan to plan even within the same MCC, so don't assume anything until you've asked. That's why you should call the insurance company/MCC as soon as possible before seeing the client so that you really know what the benefits are. Clients have a hard time understanding the issues and don't know what to ask.

Then, the client and the case manager contact the provider. The MCC authorizes a limited number of visits, for example, 3 to 10 for the clinician to assess the client and begin treatment. The case manager then sends a form which states that the sessions are indeed pre-authorized. Without this prior authorization, the services will not be paid for. If the client sees a therapist before contacting the MCC, or if he/she sees someone who is not a provider within the network, then reimbursement will either be reduced or as is most common, it will not be forthcoming. Therefore, it is essential that after a client calls in for service you have them contact their MCC before actually seeing you. Within a week or two, the MCC will send you forms that include a case history, treatment plan, goals for therapy, and client release of information forms. You must fill these out as soon as possible to ensure successful reimbursement. A good reference for report writing is Hollis's and Donn's *Psychological Report Writing*.[21]

When you get down to the last one or two sessions, you need to contact the case manager again and ask for further authorization of sessions. They will ask you if you are making progress and why you think that the client still needs to see you.

If You Need More Sessions

Some MCCs will only give you 10 sessions in all, others may go up to 30 (authorizing 10 at a time). Rarely will they give you more than this. If the client still requires long-term therapy, then you may use the medical part of their insurance, but usually at a reduced fee.

For example, after determining medical necessity (they'll send you another form to fill out), one plan under Blue Cross's MCC (Behavioral Health Access) will pay $25.00 per visit and it will no longer be case managed. Therefore, you don't need to fill out any more forms, and there isn't a numerical limit to the number of sessions, just a yearly dollar limit. Most MCCs though, say that the client must pay out of pocket. They are extremely dedicated to short-term brief therapies—the fewer sessions, the better. Even though they seem to promise 50 sessions a year, for example, the client has a very hard time ever getting those services. It's like pulling teeth sometimes. It's frustrating too that you may have an inexperienced clinician managing the case who doesn't understand the need for long-term therapy. Many case managers are BSN nurses, social workers, and marriage, family, and child counselors, but occasionally you'll have a psychologist as one. Try always to be polite, professional, and treat them with respect. Diplomacy is always warranted. Remember, they hold the key to your client's ability get help and your ability to get paid.

BILLING TIPS

Always remember when billing to include a *copy* of the authorization form that they sent you when sending in the bill (see Tables 4.6 and 4.7 sample billing forms). *Never* send in the original; they often get lost or separated from your bill. This will really speed things up though when they are processing your claim (sometimes the authorization doesn't get into the computer before your bill gets processed).

Occasionally you will need to fax or send them another copy just in case they lost yours. Also, check the dates on your form and make sure that they match the ones on your bill. Once you've done a case or two, it really isn't so hard. It's mostly frustrating though to you and your client because the MCC makes it difficult to get sessions, and they often make mistakes in processing your claims. Some MCCs take longer to get reimbursement because they first have to process your claim, and then they send it to the insurance company for payment. Others, like Behavioral Health Access (Blue Cross) are usually very quick.

Remember, the first time you bill, it will take the longest to get paid while they put you into the computer as a vendor. Don't shy away from Managed Care, though because more and more insurance companies are going to Managed Care, and most likely all of them will eventually. Instead of giving you carte blanche services as a regular insurance, they are trying to decrease their costs by overseeing the services. There is a new trend in all third-party reimbursement—the use of electronic claim processing. For information, you may contact: Health Communications Services, 10128 West Broad Street, Glen Allen, VA 23060, (800) 543-6711.

PREFERRED PROVIDER ORGANIZATIONS

The following are the 10 largest corporate PPO chains in the United States: Blue Cross-Blue Shield Association, USA HealthNet, HealthCare Compare, Private HealthCare Systems, Metropolitan Life (MetraHealth), Community Care Network, Transport Life, Traveler's Insurance, Aetna Choice Health, and Prudential Insurance. Together, they service over 16 million employees.

Becoming Part of a Managed Care/PPO Network

Now, let's talk about how to become a preferred provider within these networks. I am working with about 20 managed care/PPOs to try to have them accept PMHNs and to be a part of their organizations. So far, 11 of those that I have contacted are willing to accept PMHNs, but some are already closed in many southern California areas. Being closed means that they are not accepting any new providers and applications because: 1) there are enough providers in a particular geographical area already, and/or 2) they do not accept PMHNs as providers.

I have already discussed with the provider relations department of many California-based managed care companies what a PMHN is, the laws and insurance codes, and other pertinent information. (Please see Table 4.4 for the listings with a + [plus sign] before them; these have already been contacted and are accepting nurses in their networks.) The others haven't been contacted yet. Nearly every week, I hear back from a managed care company and am being accepted on an ongoing basis.

As soon as you can, you must start to contact the MCCs for applications to become part of their network (for a partial listing, please see Table 4.4). For a sample letter to send to MCCs, see Table 4.2. They will usually tell you that they will send you one. However, be prepared. These applications are usually lengthy and detailed. Some companies also require you to pay a fee to process their applications. I would not join one that charges.

You must have three references, and you must carry between $1,000,000 and $3,000,000 malpractice insurance. I prefer to get my malpractice insurance from TransAmerican Specialty Insurance (see below). Prices range from $128 to $350 a year and include self-employed and employed status. They delineate between NPs and CNSs. The main malpractice carrier that gives discounts through the American Nurses Association or the Psychiatric Nurses Association is:

Maginnis and Associates, P.O. Box 92450, Chicago, IL 60690, (312) 427-1441, ext. 105.

Call ANA for possible others.

When applying to the MCC provider panel, you must send in the application and also attach a copy of your license, certification, malpractice, and a resume. Some want detailed case histories. It is helpful to write about a successful short-term case that you have had and save on computer to use over and over again. Try to send a copy of the laws, the fact sheet on CNSs, a brochure and business card, and a cover letter is very important. *Always* make a copy for your files in case yours is lost and for future reference. Note the date when you sent it in and follow up if you don't hear back within 60–90 days.

It's amazing how long it takes them to process an application. Make sure that you contact your references so that they will fill out their forms and return them if necessary in a timely manner. If they refuse you because they say that they are full in your area, write another letter in three to six months.

Sometimes these MCCs will have openings which last only a short time, so don't give up. If they refuse you because of your license (rarely

happens if you send all of the documentation to them), then call the
Provider Relations Department and talk to the director about it (see Table
4.5). Finally, it may be that they are full and have a glut of providers in
your area (especially Southern California), so just go on and try with the
other companies. It is still advisable to write to them every six months
or so. Complaints about the MCCs in California can be made to: Mr.
Jerry Todd, Department of Corporations, Consumer Complaint Unit/
Health Care Service Plans, 600 South Commonwealth Avenue, Los
Angeles, CA 90005, (213) 736-3104. For others states, please contact the
local or state Department of Corporations or Insurance Commissioner.

What They Pay

Be sure that if you do contract with PPOs that you carefully read the
contract that they send. Make sure that you can agree with their terms,
and that it is congruent with your scope of practice. Don't be afraid to
ask for legal counsel. Remember the fees that you receive from Managed
Care will be lower than your usual fees.

The range for Master's-prepared clinicians seems to be $35 to $70,
with an average of $60.00. Their fees are usually based on a percentage
(5%–60%) of the Usual and Customary Reasonable Fee for your area
(UCR).[22] The fees have been going up because of the complaints from
therapists. Be aware, though, that after you terminate with their MCC,
most clients prefer to stay on with their therapist and are willing to pay
out-of-pocket to you. Some MCCs require that you give the client three
references so that they may choose others for themselves. Even at a
reduced rate, I think it behooves you to try to get on as many PPOs as
you can. Try to be flexible.

Those of you in non-Metropolitan areas, and especially those outside
of Southern California, will have an easier time getting on because in
Southern California the networks are very full. The new trend will be for
the MCCs to contract with groups of providers rather than individual
therapists. Even if you are in a private practice, you can band loosely
with other therapists to cross-refer and to apply as a group to the MCC.
Remember, to work well with Managed Care, you must be willing to
accept limited fees, work at more short-term-oriented therapy, be willing
to discuss the client's case with the case manager, and deal effectively
with utilization review.

EMPLOYEE ASSISTANCE PROGRAMS

A good idea is to develop your own Employee Assistance Programs (EAP)
to local businesses (both small and large). There does seem to be a trend

for companies to begin to contract directly with providers and bypass the managed care dilemma. As in any marketing strategy, do your homework first, maybe even talk to the Occupational Nurse to see what are the common health-illness issues for the group. Then, develop a specialty service to them, particularly preventive services. Be prepared to offer group rates. Get together with Human Resources and discuss how your services will be both cost-effective and high quality.

Some companies will pay a flat fee on a yearly basis, to cover a limited number of sessions per client, for example, 10 per year. Others will contract with you on a fee-for-services basis. Again, don't be too shy to go to small businesses and offer your services. Be sure to let them know which PPOs or HMOs with which you are currently contracted. Be willing to offer free and paid workshops, conferences, and seminars, not only to the employees, but also to the management.

Some good topics are Stress in the Workplace, How to Deal With the Difficult Employee, and How to Assess for Substance Abuse. Also, be willing to work evenings and weekends to accommodate the working client.

To become a certified EAP practitioner, you may take an exam offered by the Professional Testing Corporation. You may send for an application to: Employee Assistance Certification Commission (EACC), 4601 North Fairfax Drive, Suite 1001, Arlington, VA 22203.

NOTES

1. American Nurses Association. (1993, February). *American Nurse, 2.*
2. Sebastian, 7.
3. California Board of Registered Nursing. (1988). *Nursing Practice Act: With rules and regulations.* Sacramento: Department of Consumer Affairs.
4. California State. (1982). Insurance Codes. Sacramento, CA. Author.
5. California State. (1975). Health & Safety Codes. Sacramento, CA. Author.
6. Leslie, D. (1988). *Insurance compensation manual.* San Diego: California Association of Marriage and Family Therapists.
7. Ibid.
8. American Nurses Association/California Nurses Association. (1992). Nursing Reimbursement Conference. Appendix K.
9. *Psychotherapy Finances, 2.*
10. American Association for Marriage and Family Therapy. (1992, April). *Family therapy news.* Washington, DC: Author, p. 21.
11. American Nurses Association. (1993). *Capital Update 11* (20), Washington, DC: Author, p. 6.

12. Health Care Financing Administration. (1992, July). *Medicaid Bureau*. Baltimore, MD: Author.
13. American Psychiatric Nurses Association. (1994). *APNA News 6* (3). Washington, DC: Author, p. 8.
14. American Nurses Association. Manual on Insurance Reimbursement. Appendix A, 5.
15. California Nurses Association. (1992). *California Nurse*. San Francisco: Author.
16. American Psychiatric Association. (1994). *Diagnostic and statistical manual of mental disorders* (4th ed.). Washington, DC: Author.
17. American Psychiatric Association. (1987). *Quick reference to the diagnostic criteria from DSM-III-R*. Washington, DC: Author.
18. Webb, L., diClemente, C., Johnstone, E., Sanders, J., & Perley, R. (Eds.). (1981). *DSM III training guide*. New York: Bruner/Mazel.
19. Carpenito, L. (1992). *Nursing diagnosis: Application to clinical practice* (4th ed.). Philadelphia: J. B. Lippencott Co.
20. Aromando, L. (1989). *Mental health and psychiatric nursing*. Springhouse, PA: Springhouse Corp.
21. Hollis, J., & Donn, P. (1989). *Psychological report writing: Theory and practice*. Muncie, NY: Accelerated Development.
22. Ridgeway Financial Institute. (1992). *Managed care handbook*, 69. Jupiter, Florida: Author.

SUMMARY OF STATE EDUCATIONAL AND PRACTICE REQUIREMENTS FOR ADVANCED PRACTICE NURSING

SUMMARY IN BRIEF

All states legislatively recognize advanced practice except for Illinois, Minnesota, Pennsylvania, and Tennessee. Despite this, APNs may practice anyway in these states under expanded roles from a broad Nurse Practice Act. Fourteen states now have accredited PMHN NP programs. (See Appendix D for a listing.)

Independent Practice

APNs may work completely independently of physicians in the following states:

Alaska	Indiana	Oregon
Arizona	Maine	Rhode Island
Colorado	Maryland	South Carolina
Connecticut	Michigan	Texas
Delaware	Montana	Utah
District of Columbia	New Hampshire	Vermont
Hawaii	New Mexico	Virginia

Kansas   North Dakota   Washington
Iowa   Oklahoma   West Virginia

Scope of Practice

There are 20 states where APNs have complete autonomy over their
practice. This includes: independent practice setting, BRN statutes that
recognize APNs (including CNSs), prescriptive privileges, and the ability
to be reimbursed by third-party payors (including legislation). They are:

Alaska   Massachusetts*   Rhode Island*
Arizona   Montana   South Carolina*
Colorado   New Hampshire   Texas*
Connecticut*   New Mexico   Utah*
Delaware   North Dakota   Vermont*
District of Columbia   Oklahoma   West Virginia*
Iowa   Oregon

*These states have minimal physician involvement with prescriptive privi-
  leges, i.e., protocols, collaboration, or written guidelines. Despite this,
  APNs may still practice in independent settings.

CNSs

Most states legislatively recognize NPs, CRNSs, CNMs, and CNSs. The
states that do not define or recognize CNSs are: California, Idaho, Illinois,
Michigan, Mississippi, Nebraska, New York, North Carolina, Oregon,
Pennsylvania, and Tennessee. CNSs may practice despite this in California, Michigan, Oregon, and Tennessee. Some states recognize only psychiatric CNSs. They are: Florida, Georgia, Maryland, Massachusetts,
Minnesota, Nevada, New Hampshire, Vermont, and Washington.[1] California calls them PMHNs.

Prescriptive Privileges

All states allow for prescriptive privileges for APNs (not necessarily all
types) except for Illinois and Ohio. Some states do mandate that APNs
have physician supervision or collaboration when utilizing prescriptive
privileges, even if their practice is autonomous otherwise. Please contact
your BRN for specific prescriptive privilege guidelines. Ohio allows for

prescriptive privileges under physician supervision, protocols, and only in specified university pilot projects.

The following four states also mandate malpractice insurance for the APN who elects to practice with prescriptive privileges:[2,3] Florida, Mississippi, Wisconsin, and Wyoming. DEA numbers are available in 24 states:[4]

Alaska	Montana	Pennsylvania
Arizona	Nebraska	Rhode Island
Connecticut	Nevada	South Carolina
District of Columbia	New Hampshire	Utah
Iowa	New Mexico	Vermont
Maine	New York	Washington
Maryland	North Carolina	West Virginia
Massachusetts	North Dakota	Wisconsin
Minnesota	Oregon	Wyoming

Prescriptive privileges allow for nurses to write a prescription for noncontrolled and controlled drugs depending on regulations. Controlled substances under the DEA include Schedule (II-V), the lower number having the greatest risk of abuse/dependence.[5,6] Noncontrolled or legend drugs are other medicines, i.e., antibiotics, cardiac medications, insulin, etc. The following fifteen states allow for prescriptive authority to APNs, excluding controlled substances: Alabama, California (LP), Florida (LP), Idaho (LP), Hawaii, Kansas, Kentucky (LP), Louisiana, Michigan, Mississippi, Missouri, Nevada, New Jersey, Tennessee, and Texas.

Thirty-eight states allow prescriptive privileges for CNSs:

Alaska	Kentucky	Oklahoma
Arizona	Louisiana	Pennsylvania (LP)
Arkansas	Maine	South Carolina
Colorado	Massachusetts	Tennessee
Connecticut	Michigan	Texas
Delaware	Minnesota	Utah
District of Columbia	Missouri	Vermont
Florida	Montana	Virginia
Hawaii	Nevada	Washington
Indiana	New Hampshire	Wisconsin
Iowa	New Jersey	West Virginia
Georgia	New Mexico	Wyoming
Kansas	North Dakota	

The following states allow for prescriptive privileges for APNs, excluding

CNSs: Alaska, California, Idaho, Maryland, Mississippi, Nebraska, New York, North Carolina, Oregon, Rhode Island, and South Dakota.

Third-Party Reimbursement

Twenty-one states do not have legislative mandates for third-party reimbursement, excluding MediCaid and/or MediCare reimbursement. They are: Alabama, Arkansas, District of Columbia, Georgia, Hawaii, Idaho, Illinois, Kansas, Kentucky, Louisiana, Missouri, Nebraska, New York, Ohio, Oklahoma, Pennsylvania, South Carolina, Texas, Vermont, Utah, and Wisconsin (LP). Each state summary delineates MediCaid and/or MediCare coverage.

Reimbursement Legislation

There are 30 states that have specific legislation in place or pending that assist with third-party reimbursement for APNs. Not all types of APNs are listed in each of these insurance laws. Some only have legislative assistance for MediCaid and/or MediCare. And even though the mandates exist, there is almost universal difficulty for APNs to become part of managed care panels (PPOs, EAPs, and HMOs). Also, these mandates do not always ensure reimbursement from the other types of payors (private indemnity, self-insured, Blue Cross/Blue Shield, MediCaid, and MediCare). Most BRNs do not have much information regarding this. The following nine states are reporting that APNs are being reimbursed and included in managed care systems: Arizona, California, Florida, Kansas (LP), Kentucky, Maryland, Mississippi, New Hampshire, and North Dakota (LP). The main barrier to APN reimbursement from managed care companies is that laws are written too narrowly, and most managed care companies do not have to follow the state's insurance codes. Instead, they fall under the jurisdiction of the Department of Corporations. Many states have anti-discrimination and anti-trade language in their Insurance laws and Health & Safety Codes, yet managed care seems to be without accountability in this area. For a thoughtful article on APNs and managed care, please see Marcia Lepler's, "Managed care brings APNs mixed blessings."[7,8] All advanced practice nurses must join together to ensure a place in managed care or they will find that all of the successes in advancing nursing will be overshadowed by the lack of availability to patients and communities because they cannot be reimbursed for their services. Despite the managed care issues, the following 30 states do have specific legislation in place or pending that assist with third-party reimbursement for APNs. Almost nothing is written into these laws mandating that managed care be included.

The states are:

Alaska	Massachusetts	North Dakota
Arizona	Michigan	Oregon
California	Minnesota	Rhode Island
Colorado	Mississippi	South Dakota
Connecticut	Montana	Tennessee (LP)
Delaware	Nevada	Virginia
Florida	New Hampshire	Washington
Iowa (LP)	New Jersey	West Virginia
Maine	New Mexico	Wisconsin (LP)
Maryland	North Carolina	Wyoming

SUMMARY BY STATE

The following is an alphabetical, state by state summary of educational and practice requirements. The information was gathered by this author independently through a research questionnaire in early 1995 and updated in September 1996. They were filled out by each State Board of Nursing (usually the Executive Director or Nurse Consultant for the BRN). They have the final say over what is legal in each state. These will most likely change over time, so please check with your SBRN on an ongoing basis to keep current. Although every effort has been made to be current and accurate, this author is not responsible for changes in existing law, or for governing policies concerning APN scope of practice.

ANP	Advanced Nurse Practitioner
APN	Advanced Practice Nurse
APRN	Advanced Practice Registered Nurse
AR	Administrative Rule
ARN	Advanced Registered Nurse
ARNP	Advanced Registered Nurse Practitioner
BRN	Board of Registered Nursing
CEU	Continuing Education Unit
CNM	Certified Nurse Midwife
CNP	Certified Nurse Practitioner
CNS	Clinical Nurse Specialist

CRNA	Certified Registered Nurse Anesthetists
CS	Certified Specialist
DEA	Drug Enforcement Agency
FNP	Family Nurse Practitioner
HB	House Bill
LNM	Licensed Nurse Midwife
MSN	Master's of Science degree in Nursing
NPA	Nurse Practice Act
NM	Nurse Midwife
NP	Nurse Practitioner
PMHN	Psychiatric Mental Health Nurse
PNP	Pediatric Nurse Practitioner
RN	Registered Nurse
RNA	Registered Nurse Anesthetist
R & R	Rules and Regulations
SB	Senate Bill
SBRN	State Board of Registered Nursing

Alabama

The BRN had provided rules and regulations that recognize NPs, CNMs, CNSs, and CRNAs (see AC 610X-90.08). These ARNPs must collaborate and consult with a physician.

A bill authorizing prescriptive privileges for all APNs was introduced into legislation in 1994, and became effective July 1, 1996. This bill allows only CRNPs and CNMs to prescribe noncontrolled substances if they have a collaborating physician to countersign.

Third-party reimbursement was attempted by legislative action in 1986, but failed. Medicaid reimbursement is available to FNPs and PNPs. An insurance company, Mutual Assurance which provides up to 80% of the state's nonhospital doctors refuses to insure any physician who ''precepts'' NPs unless the doctor provides on-site supervision. This insurance company is sponsored by the Alabama Medical Association. CRNAs have specific legislation (1989) to assist with third-party reimbursement.

Alaska

There are currently 240 Licensed Advanced Nurse Practitioners (ANP) in Alaska. They include NPs, CNMs, CNSs, and CRNAs and they must meet national certification requirements. Many are referred to as CNSs or Mental Health NPs and are required to have a master's degree in nursing related to mental health. They may perform counseling services and work independently of physicians although they must have a plan for consultation and referral in place.

Independent prescriptive privileges are available after having had 15 contact hours in pharmacology within two years of initial ANP license (including Schedule II-V drugs) as long as they have a plan for physician consultation. For renewal, the nurse must maintain national certification and have eight hours of continuing education. APNs may also obtain DEA numbers.

ANPs may bill for third-party payment by Alaska insurance statutes (see 21.36.090). This statute says that there shall be no discrimination for a provider of service as long as he or she is operating under their respective scope of legal practice (including ARNPs). Despite this, some ARNPs still have some difficulty with reimbursement (mainly lack of knowledge of scope of practice by insurance companies). Medicaid reimbursement is available at 80% of physician's rates for PNPs and FNPs. Attitudes are generally healthy from other medical providers, although there has been some concern over prescriptive privileges. Doctors are being educated about this and so the situation is getting better.

Arizona

Arizona registers about 776 NPs, NMs, and CRNAs. The Rules and Regulations concerning CNSs will most likely be completed by September, 1996. They will then be certified by the state. Psychiatric mental health CNSs and psychiatric NPs are able to practice and perform counseling/psychotherapy services if educated to do so. NPs must have graduated from an NP program and be certified. NPs may work in independent practice, but must have a collaborating physician for consultation and referral.

Full prescriptive and dispensing privileges are available (see Rule 4-19-504). This includes Schedule II-V drugs.

Chapters 20-841.03, 20-1376.03, and 20-1406.03 of the Insurance Code prohibit denial of reimbursement to RNs and NPs. NPs are able to be listed on managed care contracts. CNSs have some difficulty getting third-party reimbursement. There is no provision for Medicaid reimbursement. In lieu of Medicaid, there is the Arizona Health Care Cost Containment System (AHCCS), which does contract with some NPs directly. Currently, they are reimbursed at 60% of physician rates, but there are attempts being made to increase it to 80%. Medicare reimburses NPs in rural areas only at the rate of 80% of physician reimbursement. Physician support is both positive and negative for APNs.

Arkansas

Under ACT 409, APNs are licensed in Arkansas. There are 866 registered nurse practitioners, 260 certified registered nurse anesthetists, and 10 certified nurse midwives. In 1995, CNSs were added via House Bill 1488. CNSs must be trained at the graduate level and be nationally certified. NPs must also be nationally certified and must work in collaboration with and under the direction of a physician *or* under the direction of protocols developed with a doctor. Collaborative practice must include a written plan that outlines procedures for consultation with or referral to the doctor. CRNAs must work in the presence and under the supervision of a doctor or dentist and must also be nationally certified. CNMs must work in a health care system that provides for consultation, collaborative management, or referral. They must also be nationally certified. The following titles are protected by law: APN, ARNP, CRNA, CNM, LNM, RNP, and CNS.

Prescriptive authority is granted to APNs who have a BRN approved advanced pharmacology course, completed a preceptorship, and have a collaborative practice agreement with a licensed physician. This agreement must be filed with the BRN. Prescriptive privileges are limited to Schedule III-V.

APNs may receive direct reimbursement for Medicaid programs at an 80% rate. Medicare reimbursement is also available. Some individual insurance companies do reimburse RNs. The BRN recommends legal counsel prior to setting up an independent practice as a PMHN.

California

The BRN certifies NPs (5,984), CRNAs (1,480), and CNMs (721), but not CNSs at present. CNMs and CRNAs actually get a separate license beyond the initial RN license. There are currently 255,000 RNs in California, and research from the BRN in 1994 showed that between 3% and 10% (7,650–25,000) of these RNs self-identified themselves as CNSs.[9] Most nurses with master's degrees in nursing call themselves CNSs; the term is not protected by law, but will most likely be in 1998. And of course, those nurses who are ANCC certified, as CNSs, do use the term regardless of education. The BRN has taken the position that a licensed registered nurse may perform counseling services without any additional licensing or certification. Psychiatric mental health nurses, as they are called in California, may work independently and may bill for third-party payments without being listed by the BRN. Currently, there are about

450 such nurses listed with the BRN. All nurses, even APNs, work under the same scope of practice. Generally, a PMHN is a nurse with a master's degree in nursing directly related to mental health with two years of supervised experience. These nurses may be listed with the BRN for ease in insurance reimbursement. This listing is not mandatory and does not alter the scope of nursing practice. Nurses with master's degrees in related fields may do counseling work under the same scope of practice as these PMHNs, and may also use the term PMHN. Both may be in private practice and work independently of physicians. The other types of APNs must work under "standardized procedures," which is a collaborative relationship with a physician; the level of supervision varies with practice site. The PMHN with an MSN meets insurance code requirements and can receive third-party reimbursement more easily than those nurses with master's degrees other than in nursing, for instance, counseling. No matter what, you must be trained to do the services that you perform. Since psychotherapy is a skill taught at the master's level, this is the expected level of educational preparation.

There is a distinction between the kind of counseling a (bachelor's in nursing) RN can do and the psychotherapy that a master's-level nurse can do. The BRN at this time has not specified which kind of education you need, but they seem to support a master's degree in psychiatric nursing and two years of supervised experience.

You need to contact them for specific information about how the Nurse Practice Act affects you and the particular education and experience requirements.[10] There are specific guidelines for nurse practitioners, but not for clinical nurse specialists at present. The BRN hopes to regulate CNSs by 1998. About 2,200 NPs may have prescriptive privileges called "furnishing licenses" under physician protocols. They may apply for DEA numbers. CNMs also have this authority. They both qualify for it if they have postgraduate training in pharmacology, completed six months of supervised experience, and have an ongoing supervising physician. A new bill (AB1077) passed in September 1996 allows NPs to furnish medical devices and Schedule III-V drugs under protocols with a supervising physician.[11,12]

The BRN will certify CNSs just like they do with the other three types of APNs. In 1994, Assembly Bill 518 passed which mandated that the BRN study the role of the CNS in order to establish legislation to protect the title "CNS," and to set educational and practice standards. A survey was done in September 1994 which polled over 210,000 California nurses and over 1,000 responded who see themselves as CNSs. The BRN reported back to the legislation in December 1994 to discuss the results of the research and to establish legislation that will most likely take effect in

1998. The bill is currently in the Senate and may pass in 1997 and become law January 1, 1998. The BRN will likely establish regulations in 1997. A preliminary report was sent to me by the BRN and they are taking the stand that clinical nurse specialists must be certified (hopefully in 1998). They will require a master's degree in nursing with a clinical specialty, since this is the national trend and the professional standard. Also, almost 70% of the nurses polled had MSN preparation. The BRN *will not* require ANA certification because there are only a few specialty exams available. Possibly in the future, they will require certification if an exam exists in all CNS clinical specialties. They will be grandfathering in those nurses with advanced degrees in related fields (probably for a limited time). This provision is especially referring to school nurses and PMHNs with master's degrees in counseling, etc. The research showed that nurses with master's degrees outside of nursing were older and had more experience in nursing (over 15% of those surveyed were in this category). I believe that this reflects the fact that there were few MSN programs 15 to 20 years ago and so nurses were forced to seek graduate education in related fields. Now there seem to be plenty of graduate programs in nursing available in California.

The main barriers to PMHN/CNS practice cited in the BRN report were as follows: lack of admitting privileges, lack of direct reimbursement, lack of recognition of the CNS in the Nurse Practice Act, lack of recognition or understanding of the CNS role, physicians' fear of competition, perception of physicians as "captain of the ship," NPs being favored over CNSs, and limited ability to write orders in hospitals.

If you are a California CNS, please keep in contact with the BRN for these changes. MediCal (Medicaid) reimbursement is available for FNPs, PNPs, NPs, CRNAs, and CNMs. MediCare reimbursement is available to APNs, including CNSs in rural areas only. California, like many states, seems to be writing all of their legislation for nurses with master's degrees in nursing only, and omitting others. Even when CNSs are certified, I don't think that nurses with master's degrees in counseling and related fields will be excluded from practice because of the grandfathering clause. The last thing we need to do is to exclude these advanced practice nurses because they have a degree outside of nursing, especially if they are ANCC certified as CNSs. Even though the national current trend is to do away with the confusion over clinical nurse specialists and nurse practitioners, especially now since all are master's-degree prepared, California will keep the distinction. It is difficult for many nurses, medical professionals, and the public to understand the various titles. Again, the move nationally seems to be to have a new title: Advanced Practice RN (APRN) or Advanced Registered Nurse Practitioner (ARNP). For your interest, please contact the BRN and they will send you their position paper on the "Scope of the PMHN in California."

Listing with the CBRN/PMHN Number

California has specific legislation in the Insurance Codes that mandate direct reimbursement for psychiatric mental-health registered nurses (see Insurance Codes 10176, 10176.7, 10177, 10177.8, 11512.3 at end of chapter 1).[13] (Please also review Table 4.5.) These laws also include the services of a licensed psychologist, licensed clinical social worker, and a marriage family and child counselor. These laws say that RNs who have master's degrees in nursing and two years of supervised experience must be reimbursed by third-party payors as defined within if the plan covers mental-health services. It also mandates that the Board of Registered Nursing keep a listing of such nurses.

This does not mean that a psychiatric mental-health nurse must be listed with the BRN in order to bill insurance companies. Nor does it mean that PMHNs with master's degrees in counseling cannot bill insurance companies either. As long as the nurse may legally perform the services, she is entitled to bill directly. Many nurses either do not know about this listing or refuse to do it.

In order to be listed with the BRN, the nurse must make an application for a PMHN number, have a master's degree in nursing in a field directly related to mental health, and have verification of two years of supervised experience or be certified as a psychiatric clinical specialist by the American Nurses Credentialing Center. Currently, certified clinical nurse specialists with master's degrees in counseling or marriage and family therapy may not be listed or receive a PMHN number, but their scope of practice is neither limited nor expanded in any way because of this. For all intents and purposes, there is no difference. Hopefully, CNSs as a wide category will be added to the Insurance Codes for ease of reimbursement. I have not had any difficulty with reimbursement because I have not been listed with the BRN.

Insurance companies are not making a distinction; they do seem to want the RN to be certified though as a specialist and have a master's degree. I do encourage you though to apply for listing and receive a PMHN number because it will make your case for insurance reimbursement stronger. It may also be that in the future, insurance companies will be more strict about wanting the nurse to have this number. But remember, the law does not say that you must have this number or be listed to receive insurance monies.

Finally, when billing please be sure to include this PMHN number after your credentialing information. You may also want to include a photocopy of this certificate along with your license, when sending information about yourself to insurance companies.

Evidence Code

In 1992, Psychiatric Mental Health Nurses with two years of supervised experience were added to Section 1010(8) of the Evidence Code by way of California Assembly Bill 3035. This Code is used to allow for Patient-Psychotherapist privilege and allows for confidentiality for a PMHN, physician, psychologist, licensed clinical social worker, marriage, family and child counselor, and a psychologist assistant or registered MFCC intern or social worker assistant or trainee.

Even though nurses have always respected confidentiality and it is within our *Code of Ethics*, this still is a victory for us legally.[14] An essential boon for us in California is that insurance companies use the Evidence Code when writing their policies in determining who is a "psychotherapist." Even though this is not a legal definition, they still go by it.

Colorado

Under Rules and Regulations, Chapter 14, APNs may practice in Colorado. CNMs, CNAs, and NPs must be nationally certified. CNSs must have a master's or doctoral degree in a clinical nursing specialty. National certification is not mandated. The titles APN, CNM, CNS, CRNA, and NP are protected under law (see 12-38-111.5). After July 1, 1995, all APNs must complete national accreditation or certification. After July 1, 2008, all APNs must have completed a graduate degree within their specialty.

Since January 1996, prescriptive privileges, including controlled substances (Schedule IV-V) are available for all APNs under Chapter 15 of the Rules and Regulations of the Nurse Practice Act. To qualify, the nurse must be listed on the BRN registry, have a graduate degree in a nursing specialty, have coursework in the use of prescription and controlled drugs, and have postgraduate training of at least 1800 hours (in the previous 5 yrs). All APNs who are listed on the BRN advanced practice registry will receive an application for prescriptive privileges. Those APNs with prescriptive authority must also have a written collaborative agreement with a physician, but they do not need to be directly supervised by one. The NPA should be read in detail for a complete understanding of the requirements (see 12–38–111.6).

RNs may bill for third-party reimbursement subject to 12-38-128 of the NPA which says that nurses cannot be prohibited from such billing.

There is no specific legislation to assist with reimbursement. No provision for Medicare has been made. PNPs, FNPs, CNMs and CRNAs have been able to receive Medicaid reimbursement at 100% of physician's fees. The only recognized involvement for managed care is case management. The obvious barrier to practice here is the limitation of nurses to advance practice by the obvious lack of legislative definitions and guidelines.

Connecticut

Nationally certified clinical specialists and nurse practitioners are allowed to engage in advanced practice with their RN license. CRNAs and NMs require a special ARNP license to practice. Also, if the CS/NP is prescribing, dispensing, and diagnosing, then they must also have this secondary license. The Psychiatric CS/NP may use the terms counseling and psychotherapy. The educational requirements for all four types of advanced practice is national certification by the appropriate board. If the nurse was certified after 1994, then he or she must possess a master's degree in nursing.

All ARNPs must have a directing physician for practice and prescriptive authority (including Schedule II-V drugs). They must have completed a 30-hour course in pharmacology. They may also apply for independent DEA numbers.

They are able to bill for third-party payment, but their reimbursement rates are lower than that of physicians. There is some difficulty getting on managed care panels/Health Maintenance Organizations. There are specific laws assisting reimbursement for nurses. Please contact the Department of Insurance for a copy. No Medicare reimbursement is available, and Medicaid reimbursement to FNPs and PNPs is currently being determined. The main barriers to practice are the physician supervision requirement and managed care difficulties.

Delaware

ARNPs are recognized here. Legislation passed in 1994 that divided them into NPs, CNSs, CNMs, and CRNAs. They must have a year of postgraduate education and be nationally certified. If no national exam is available, then they must have a master's degree. Thirteen separate categories of ARNPs are granted practice including five CNS specialties.

In 1994, legislation introduced HB 274 which provides for full prescriptive authority for ARNPs. Since January 1996, they may prescribe Schedule II-V drugs under a collaborative agreement with a physician. They must apply for their own DEA number.

In 1991, the Insurance Codes were amended to mandate reimbursement for ARNPs if the provider is within their respective scope of practice. FNPs and PNPs receive Medicaid reimbursement at 100% of physician's fees.

District of Columbia

The Health Occupations Division defines NP practice and ARNPs are given a specialty certificate by the BRN. They include NPs, CNMs, and CRNAs. Psychiatric CNSs chose not to be listed as ARNs 10 years ago, but are now included on the list. Since March 1996, ARNPs can work independent of any collaboratiave agreements or protocols with a physician.

Even though there are no insurance codes that mandate reimbursement for APNs, some private payors are doing so anyway. CNMs receive 100% of physician fees under Medicaid. Psychiatric CNSs are not reimbursed by third-party payors because they are considered to be working beyond the scope of an RN.

The new law changes this. APNs are receiving direct reimbursement if providing mental health care, including alcohol/drug abuse counseling. All APNs have full prescriptive authority (Schedule II-V). The Board of Pharmacy did not initially approve of this, but has been providing DEA numbers since October, 1995. MediCaid is available to physicians only. NPs can be reimbursed by private insurance companies.

Florida

NPs, CNMs, CRNAs and Psychiatric CNSs are certified as ARNPs by the BRN. They must all work under physician protocols. They may work in private practice if they have a doctor who sponsors them. Legislation was introduced in 1994 (FS 464) that would delete physician supervision/ protocols and would add CNSs (all types) to the list of ARNPs but failed.

In 1988, NPs gained prescriptive privileges (no controlled substances). ARNPs prescribe under protocols with their attending physician. In May of 1996, a bill was approved by the Senate that would 1) study giving ARNPs prescriptive authority for controlled substances, increase educational standards for CRNAs, NPs and Psychiatric CNSs, allow for APNs to order diagnostic tests and physical therapy, and allow for CNMs and CRNAs to be provisionally certified after graduation, but before national certification exams. The results of this study are due back to the legislature by December 31, 1997. Hopefully, the bill willl pass then, or early 1998 and become effective 1998-9.[15] All ARPNs with prescriptive privileges are mandated to carry malpractice insurance.

ARNPs receive Medicare (rural and underserved areas), Medicaid (80% fees), Champus, and all other health insurance reimbursement.

Georgia

According to the last survey, the BRN reported 664 NPs, 17 CNMs, 241 CRNAs, and 157 CNSs. The Georgia Nurse Practice Act defines advanced practice in sections 43-26-3 and Chapter 410-12. Herein lie rules and regulations for NPs, RNAs, CNMs, and CNSs (psychiatric/mental health). Only CNSs in the area of psychiatric mental-health nursing are recognized. They are given a "letter of recognition," but are not issued a license or certificate per se. The CNS must hold a master's degree or higher in nursing with a specialization in psychiatric/mental health nursing or hold current national ANA certification as a clinical specialist. Only those nurses who meet the previous qualifications may use the term CNS. These nurses may perform counseling and psychotherapy as determined by ANA standards.

There are no independent prescriptive privileges allowed, but some provision of ordering and dispensing drugs is based on written protocols using a formulary (see chapter 410-13.01).

FNPs, PNPs, OB/GYN NPs, CRNAs (all at 90%), and CNMs (100%) may receive Medicaid reimbursement. Some private insurers do reimburse ARNPs, but are not mandated to do so by law. For reimbursement issues, contact the Georgia Department of Medical Assistance (Chery Clark), (404) 656-3961.

Hawaii

The HBRN is working to specifically address advanced practice; the scope of nursing practice has previously been written very broadly. The BRN is writing legal definitions to specify advanced practice and hopes to be finished by late 1996. This same year brought new legislation which provides for prescriptive privileges for APNs and includes a formulary. The Rules and Regulations will be completed in late 1996. The BRN hopes that it will take effect by 1997. The criteria for APNs will be similar to that of Oregon. All will be considered NPs and must possess a master's degree in nursing and be certified by the ANA. Please contact the BRN in late 1996 for details.

NPs, CNSs, CRNAs, and CNM's may prescribe using a formulary, excluding controlled substances, and must be in collaboration or with a physician. Psych CNSs have a separate formulary. To obtain prescriptive privileges, these APNs must have completed 30 hours of advanced pharmacology and 1000 hours of clinical experience.

Reimbursement is improving in Hawaii. NPs are able to be reimbursed by MediCaid at 75% of physicians's fees and CHAMPUS also reimburses them as well. There is a move to insure "the uninsured", titled the "Hawaii Health Quest" which does recognize PNPs, FNPs, and CNMs as providers.[16]

Idaho

The Joint Rules with the Board of Medicine allows for the practice of nurse practitioners (see IDAPA 23, Title 01, Chapter 01). Currently, there are 126 active NPs, none of which are in private practice. The BRN broadened the scope of practice for NPs in 1991 after a bill to eliminate physician supervision was defeated. CNMs are considered NPs. CRNAs are considered separately and have their own registration. There is no recognition of CNSs. NPs may perform counseling services, but must be supervised by a physician with protocols and also for orders of medication and treatment. These NPs must have at a minimum a BSN, be trained formally as a NP, and be nationally certified. Since there is no legal recognition of CNSs, there is no requirement for ANCC certification.

Prescriptive privileges may be applied for if the NP has at least 30 hours of pharmacology training, and must be carried out via protocols with the supervising doctor. For a complete list of the approved formulary, see IDAPA 23.01.01-341). There is a revision of the formulary up for revision at present that would expand it to include Schedule III-V drugs, but it still has not passed.

There is no legislation for third-party payment. NPs have had Medicaid reimbursement capacity for years and the term NP is defined by law. Because there must be a supervisory relationship between the nurse and doctor, the fees are paid directly to the doctor at 85%.. Medicare reimbursement is also available. The main barrier is the lack of independent practice and that there is no provision for the CNS. The BRN is exploring this at present. Many physicians have been supportive of advanced practice in this state.

Illinois

The Nursing Act of 1987 (65/3L) covers advanced practice nursing within the broad definition of "professional nursing," and which includes *all its specialties.* Illinois has 110,000 RNs, but the BRN has no listing of ARNPs. There is no special title except Registered Nurse, which is protected by law. There is no special licensure or state certification, and national certification is not required. Advanced practice nurses may work independently of physicians, but must have collaboration/supervision.

There is no provision for prescriptive privileges even though it is implicit in the NPA. No specific guidelines are outlined for the various types of advanced practice.

Nor is there any legislative assistance for reimbursement except as follows. On December 22, 1993, the Attorney General issued a statement that would allow the 700 plus certified NPs to receive direct Medicaid reimbursement.[17] Since July of 1995, PNPs and FNPs receive reimbursement at 70% of the physician rate. MediCare follows the federal guidelines. Some private insurers do pay for the services of some APNs, but there is no legislative mandate for this. The main barrier is that the Nurse Practice Act is extremely broad and is not much help in defining or directing advanced practice so far.

Indiana

This state recently amended its Nurse Practice Act to recognize nurse practitioners, clinical nurse specialists, and nurse midwives as ARNPs. They are defined in Article 23, Chapter 25-23-1-1, which was developed by HB 1564 (1993). CRNAs are defined in 25-23-1-1-4 and are seen as a separate category.

The legislation also provides for prescriptive authority. The BRN, in the summer of 1994, detailed the rules and regulations governing advanced practice including educational requirements and scope of practice. The APNs will have to work collaboratively with a doctor for prescriptive privileges. The APN must complete a two-unit semester course on pharmacology, and the prescriptive authority will be limited to the scope of the supervising physician. Controlled substances (Schedule II-V) are included. APNs must obtrain BRN approval and a DEA number.

NPs may receive third-party reimbursement by insurers that want to participate. Medicare reimbursement is by federal guidelines, and Medicaid reimbursement is at 85% of the physician's fees. Please contact the BRN for up-to-date information.

Iowa

The BRN licenses Advance Practice Registered Nurses including RNAs, NPs, CNSs and NMs. This is a secondary license beyond the basic RN license. All of the various types of advanced practice nurses are called ARNPs, and must be nationally certified. Specifically, the "certified CNS" is considered an ARNP (see Chapter 7, p. 1 IAC). The "certified PMHN practitioner" is an ARNP with a master's degree and ANCC certification. Both must possess a master's degree in nursing directly related to mental health. Psychiatric ARNPs may perform counseling and psychotherapy services.

ARNPs may work independently of physicians and have prescriptive authority of Schedule II-V drugs (excluding CRNAs). They may also apply for their own DEA number.

Certified RNs may be reimbursed by third-party payors by law, but ARNPs are not being paid. There are plans to introduce new reimbursement legislation in 1997. They do receive Medicaid reimbursement at the rate of 80%–100% of physician's fees. There is no provision for Medicare. One strength of this BRN is the detailed definitions and recognition of the various subspecialties of advanced practice nursing in their Nurse Practice Act.

Kansas

Advanced practice nurses are certified in Kansas and are called advanced registered nurse practitioners. The following categories may be applied for to the BRN: NP, RNA, NM, and Clinician Specialist (CS). CSs are able to perform counseling services. CSs must have a master's degree in nursing directly related to mental health; the other three ARNPs do not require master's-degree preparation. ANCC certification is not required, for the CS, but is recognized as one avenue to certification within the state. The other ARNPs must all be certified.

All ARNPs may work independently of physicians, but must work with a physician when prescribing medications (excluding most controlled substances). In this case, there must be written protocols. The BRN hoped that legislation would be passed in 1994 that would expand the authority to exclude physician supervision and add scheduled drugs. They now believe it will be a few more years yet for this to pass. Starting in January, 1997, ARNPs will be required to take a 3-hour pharmacology course. A few minor changes have improved prescriptive authority. They were able to add some scheduled drugs and make it easier to write (not always phone in) prescriptions.

ARNPs may bill for third-party payment and are getting paid at present. There is specific legislation from 1990 that mandates insurance reimbursement for ARNPs. Medicaid (at 80%–100% of doctors' fees) and Medicare reimbursement is also available. Currently, ARNPs are not included in managed care, but changes are being made in this area.

Kentucky

The KBRN registers (in the form of licensure) advanced registered nurse practitioners (ARNPs) and designates them as either a nurse anesthetist, nurse practitioner, nurse midwife, or clinical nurse specialist. There are a total of 1,072 ARNPs at this time: 709 RNAs, 65 NMs, 264 NPs, 2 CNSs, and 13 combined Psychiatric CNSs/NPs. This latter group may perform counseling services (see AOS #85-13). They must have a master's degree directly related to mental health and be certified as a CNS by the ANA. All ARNPs must have their respective national certifications. CNSs may work independently of physicians, but must act according to established protocols (see 201 KAR 20:057).

Prescriptive privileges are available via established protocols (M.D. must sign the prescription). In 1994, legislation was introduced that seeks to clarify prescriptive authority for the ARNP, but failed. The Pharmacy Board and the Attorney General do not accept this and are countering independent prescriptive privileges. ARNPs cannot obtain a DEA number. New legislation will be introduced by 1997 that will assist in promoting prescription privileges.

ARNPs may bill for third-party payment, although no specific legislation exists and all payors are not cooperative. ARNPs may be reimbursed by Medicaid (at 75% of physicians' fees) and Medicare. The Kentucky Department of Medicaid Services can be reached at: 275 E. Main St., Frankfort, KY, 40621. The Medicare Carrier is at: 100 E. Vine St., Lexington, KY, 40507. Managed care contracts are also open to CNSs. The barriers for ARNPs in Kentucky are the lack of clear statutory authority for prescriptive privileges, and lack of reimbursement by all payors.

Louisiana

On January 1, 1996 (Act 633) became effective which licenses APRNs to include: NPs, CRNA's, CNMs and CNSs. Currently, there are 595 such nurses in Louisiana; of these, nine are in private practice. All APRNs must have a master's degree in nursing. ANCC certification is not required. The CNS title is now protected by law. CNSs can be independent, but NPs and RNAs must work under the direction of a physician. CNSs may provide counseling services.

There is very limited prescriptive authority under physician-directed collaboration agreements.

There is no state legislation that assists with third-party reimbursement, and so many of the advanced practice nurses are having difficulty with third-party payors. Currently, only CRNAs, CNMs, FNPs, and PNPs may bill for Medicare and Medicaid (at 80%–100% of physicians' fees). CNSs are excluded. The main barrier to practice in this state is the prohibition against medical diagnosis and medical prescriptive authority. The BRN encourages nurses to work with the LNA to overcome these barriers through legislative action. Individual physicians often support advanced practice but organized medicine seems to oppose it.

Maine

Maine defines an advanced practice nurse (ARNPs) as a RN who holds postgraduate education from a formal program designed to train nurses for an advanced practice role and who is nationally certified. Section 2102 2B states that they may "perform acts of medical diagnosis and the prescription of medical, therapeutic, or corrective measures when delegated by a physician *or* when the nurse is authorized on the basis of specialized training as a CNA."[18]

Chapter 8 of the Rules and Regulations of the Maine State Board of Nursing clearly spells out specifics for the three types of advanced practice nurses. Clinical nurse specialists fall under section 2102 2A of the Maine nurse practice act and practice as "registered professional nurses."[19] Since January of 1996, CNSs were added to the list of ARNPs. NPs must have had an additional two years supervised experience under a physician.

Psychiatric mental-health nurses may practice counseling/psychotherapy services only if so trained. The Maine Insurance Code does spell out mandated reimbursement though for certified (ANA) clinical specialists in adult/and child psychiatric mental-health nursing. NPs are not specifically named in the codes, but many NPs will have this certification already and so will be covered.

No one may use the term "certified" unless they have specific approval by the Board.

Certified nurse practitioners and CNSs who qualify as ARNPs may "dispense or prescribe medications, by written or by verbal order," when authority to do so has been specifically delegated by a licensed primary *supervising* physician. This includes Schedule III-V drugs. They may apply for a DEA number as well.

As of 10/20/93, there were a total of 639 advanced practice nurses in Maine. Of these, 318 were nurse practitioners, 35 were certified nurse midwives, and 286 were certified registered nurse anesthetists.

Certified psychiatric CNSs are qualified for third-party reimbursement. Medicaid and Medicare reimbursement is also available for NPs and CNMs. A new law regarding MediCare should be introduced in 1996.

Maryland

The BRN recognizes CNMs, NPs, CRNAs, and nurse psychotherapists in independent practice (CSP). The last group is not considered an NP, and is defined in Title 10, chapter 12 of the NPA. There are a total of 1,825 APNs in all categories (228 CSPs). These last nurses may ''establish a mental health diagnosis, provide individual, group, and family therapy, and any therapy whose purpose is to effect client change to alleviate emotional disturbances, reverse or change maladaptive behavior, and facilitate personality growth or development.''[20] They must hold a master's degree or higher (nonspecific) and be ANCC certified. NPs must be certified by their respective boards.

The CSPs may work independently of physicians, but do not have prescriptive privileges. NPs and CNMs may prescribe in collaboration with physicians including controlled substances (Schedule II-V). They may apply for their own DEA numbers.

APNs may bill for third-party payments, but are having some difficulty with some private insurance companies even though the Maryland Insurance Codes (1987 rev.) says that any health care provider can bill for their services. The BRN is working with the Attorney General on this issue. Medicaid pays 100% to APNs. Medicare reimbursement is also available with some limitations. Medicare (Part B) reimburses CRNPs and CRNAs in designated rural areas and in skilled nursing facilities. Psychiatric mental-health nursing specialists are mentioned in the Evidence Code (see Article Courts and Judicial Procedures Section 9-109.1). APNs may be listed with managed care contracts, but there are some exclusions from private insurances and Health Maintenance Organizations. There seems to be some opposition toward the CSP from psychologists.

Massachusetts

The BRN regulates NPs, NMs, NAs, and psychiatric nurse mental health clinical specialists. There are approximately 1,800, 250, 750, and 610 of these advanced nurses, respectively. The BRN ''authorizes'' their practice, but there is no second licensure. The CNS may ''deliver mental health care which includes evaluative, diagnostic, consultative, and therapeutic procedures....'' They may use the term counseling or psychotherapy. A master's degree in counseling, psychology, or related fields is required, as is ANCC certification. Since January 1994, there has been a change to require a master's degree in nursing for new applicants. The term "CNS" is protected by law. These nurses may work independently of a physician, but must have some practice guidelines with a doctor, psychologist, licensed clinical social worker, or other CNS.

The nurse may opt for prescriptive privileges, including Schedule II-V drugs. They are allowed to apply for a DEA number. NPs, CNMs, and PCSs must work with written guidelines with a *Psychiatrist* or other physician (non-PCSs), have had 24 contact hours of training in pharmacotherapeutics, and the prescribing practice must be reviewed every three months.

These advanced practitioners may bill for third-party payments, and are not having difficulties. Specific legislation exists to reimburse CPSs, CRNAs, and CNMs. As of April 1995, legislation was passed to include reimbursement for all NPs. This law does not include HMOs or managed care plans. Medicare reimbursement is not available here. Some limited Medicaid reimbursement is available for some NPs (100% rate). The main barrier seems to be the mandated link to psychiatrists when the CNS has prescriptive privileges.

Michigan

Nurse specialty certifications are outlined in Part 4 of the Administrative Rules for the BRN. Only RNAs, CNMs, and NPs are recognized. CNSs are not so defined, but may practice anyway. Psychiatric CNSs are considered APNs. NPs must have graduated from an accredited program that prepares NPs and he or she must also be nationally certified as such in the respective specialty area.

There is no requirement for supervision or collaboration with a physician except with prescriptive privileges. Prescriptive authority is granted to the specialty nurse only under proper delegation from a physician (excluding controlled substances). A new bill sponsored by the Michigan Nurses Association would allow for independent prescriptive privileges and will be heard by the Senate in the fall of 1996.[21]

These licensed specialty nurses may not be denied by Blue Cross-Blue Shield for services rendered (at an 85% rate of doctors' fees with some limitations) as long as the law doesn't require the service to only be rendered by a physician or by direct supervision of one, for example anesthesia (Attorney General Ruling). Legislation passed in 1995 mandates third-party reimbursement to all APNs. Also, Medicare reimbursement is available to NPs, CNSs, CNMs, and CRNAs. MediCaid reimbursement is available to NPs at 100%.

Minnesota

There are no specific guidelines for advanced practice; APNs are covered under a broad NPA.

NPs and Psychiatric CNSs have prescriptive privileges (Schedule II-V) under physician delegation. CNMs have the same prescriptive privileges without physician involvement. DEA numbers are available to all APNs.

Legislative mandates are in place for third-party reimbursement for NPs, CNMs, CRNAs, and psychiatric CNSs. Most APNs are reimbursed at the 90–100% rate of physician's fees from Medicaid. No other information was available from the BRN. Please contact them with specific practice questions.

Mississippi

The BRN says that there are 577 nurse practitioners of the various subspecialties in Mississippi, but there are none in psychiatric mental health. They do recognize CRNAs, CNMs, and NPs, but not CNSs (see R&R chapter 4 of Nurse Practice Law). These advanced practice nurses may perform counseling. They must possess a BRN or higher degree in nursing and be nationally certified by their respective boards. They must work in a collaborative/consultative relationship with a physician. They must also have written protocols in place.

NPs also have prescriptive authority, with some limits on controlled substances via protocols. Malpractice insurance is mandated by the BRN if they utilize prescriptive privileges. CRNAs and CNMs may order Scheduled drugs in a licensed facility. DEA numbers are not available.

They may bill for third-party reimbursement, are getting paid, but a physician co-signature is still required. They can also bill for Medicare and Medicaid (90% of doctor's fees) services. They are also included on some managed care contracts. The BRN would recognize and allow for the practice of psychiatric NPs, but since there are few programs training psychiatric NPs, this will continue to be a barrier to practice in Mississippi unless they certify CNSs or accept their training as being equivalent to that of an NP.

Missouri

The Nursing Practice Act (335.016) recognizes advanced practice nurses. On August 28, 1993, House Bill 564 passed that relates to the collaborative practice between physicians and advanced practice nurses. It defined advanced practice nurses (335.016.[2], p.57). Under Title 4, Division 200, chapter 4, General Rules, Nurse Specialty Titles have been defined (see 4 CSR 200-4.100). These include CRNAs, CNMs, CNPs, and CNSs. This latter group must be an RN with a master's degree in the area of clinical nursing *or* be certified by the ANCC. These are all protected terms. The NPA is silent about independent practice and the BRN suggests that the nurse contact an attorney first before starting a private practice. Generally, an agreement listing protocols written with a collaborating physician is required. The board does want the nurse to have a written referral and consultation plan available also with a physician. The APN may use the term psychotherapy if she or he is so trained and acts within the scope of nursing practice.

If the nurse wishes to prescribe medicines (excluding controlled substances except by special arrangement), then there must be a collaborative practice relationship with a physician in place. They may include the authority to dispense drugs and provide treatment (see Missouri Healing Arts Practice Act, 1993).

Medicaid reimbursement is available for NPs at 100% of physician's fees. Medicare reimbursement is available for all APNs via federal guidelines. Blue Cross and Blue Shield has a nondiscriminatory policy toward APNs. Other private insurers vary in their reimbursement policies. Some new legislation is planned to assist with third-party reimbursement. MediCaid reimbursement is available to all APNs at the 100% rate.

Montana

In 1993, the NPA included coverage of CNSs in the list of advanced practice nurses. For some time, it has recognized nurse midwives, nurse practitioners, and registered nurse anesthetists. The BRN can only document 140 NPs at present. In 1994, Psychiatric CNSs were recognized and for the first time, were able to perform counseling/psychotherapy. These CNSs are required to be ANCC certified. NPs must be certified, but do not have to be master's prepared. Since June 30, 1995 CNSs getting initial certification must have a master's degree (see MOR 8.32.305).

All APNs may work independently of a physician and may have independent prescriptive authority (see MOR 8.32.1501). The latter includes controlled substances (Schedule II-V). They must have a quality assurance program in place that includes a referral process. Along with this are continuing education requirements before (15 hours) and after privileges are granted (every two years). They may also apply for DEA numbers.

ARNPs are widely being reimbursed by third-party payors. CNSs were added in 1994 to the insurance reimbursement laws to join the other three types of advanced practice nurses. Blue Cross-Blue Shield reimburses ARNPs at 80% of physician's rates. Medicaid also reimburses at this same rate. Currently, Medicare reimbursement is not an issue for these nurses. The general attitude toward advanced practice nurses has been very accepting.

Nebraska

The state of Nebraska does regulate the practice of CRNAs, CNPs, and CNMs. These three types of APRNs are certified and licensed by the state. CNSs do not have a legally expanded scope and are therefore not regulated. Currently, there are 200 CNAs, 55 CNPs, and 3 CNMs. Any registered nurse may perform counseling, and the certified NPs (psychiatric) are able to as well. They must have graduated from a program in advanced nursing, but do not need a specific degree at present. National certification is required, though. They must have a collaborative relationship with a physician and have a written practice agreement.

This is especially true in order to have prescriptive privileges which include Schedule II-V controlled substances.

These nurses may bill for third-party reimbursement, but there is no specific legislation to assist with this. CNPs are paid the same as physicians for Medicaid. Medicare reimbursement is also available per federal guidelines.

Nevada

Advanced practitioners of nursing (APNs) are certified by the BRN and must practice with a collaborating physician using standard protocols (minimum requirement is telecommunication). There are roughly 150 such NPs in Nevada. The term APN includes NPs, nurse midwives and nurse psychotherapists. CRNAs not considered APNs, can work independently and do not have prescriptive privileges. Nurse psychotherapists or APNs with a psychiatric specialty may perform counseling/psychotherapy (see NRS 632.120). They must possess a BSN and a master's degree in nursing directly related to mental health or a master's degree in counseling/psychology. ANCC certification is not required for CNSs, but certification is required of NPs. A master's degree will be required for all APNs by the year 2005. A written collaborative agreement with a physician must be submitted to the BRN for all APNs.

Prescriptive privileges are available after 1,000 hours of practice (see NAC 632.257) and through written protocols with a doctor. Controlled substances are excluded. DEA numbers are available.

There is specific legislation to assist with third-party reimbursement, but it doesn't specifically include PMHNs. NPs and CRNAs don't have difficulty with reimbursement and it is at the same rate as physicians. Medicaid reimbursement is available at 85% of physician's fees. Medicare reimburses per federal guidelines.

New Hampshire

New Hampshire recognizes advanced practice nurses and uses the initials ARNP. NPs, CNMs, CRNAs, and Psychiatric CNSs are considered APNs. There are 502 ARNPs in New Hampshire and they may work independently of physicians. Psychiatric ARNPs may perform counseling/psychotherapy. The BRN does not require ANA certification per se, but does require national certification by the board per specialty. New Hampshire regulates advanced practice by licensure.

These ARNPs may apply for prescriptive privileges including controlled (Schedule II-V) and noncontrolled substances. DEA numbers are available.

ARNPs may bill for third-party payment, but they do experience some difficulty in this area despite existing laws. ARNPs are not named in the Evidence Code. They are defined (but not CNSs) in both Medicare and Medicaid legislation and do not have any difficulty in getting reimbursement (100% of physician's fees). These nurses also have been able to become part of managed care contracts/panels. The main barrier to practice is that psychiatric ARNPs are seen as ''counselors'' and because of this have difficulty with third-party payment.

New Jersey

In 1992, legislation was introduced that mandated master's-level education for all NPs and CNSs; this bill was finalized May 2, 1994.[22] This bill, the NP/CNS Certification Act (PL 1991, Chapter 377), makes the use of these terms protected by law. These advanced practice nurses must now be graduates from a master's degree program which is designed to educate and prepare them. They must also pass the highest level exam for advanced practice, which the BRN will stipulate. There is a grandfathering clause that ended January 1, 1995, which allowed those to practice who do not have a master's degree, but who do meet the other criteria. CNMs are regulated by the Board of Medical Examiners. CRNAs are regulated by the BRN, but have no specific statutes regarding them at present.

Prescriptive privileges (excluding controlled substances) can be obtained if the applicant has successfully passed a graduate level course in pharmacology within five years of May 2, 1994. If the course is older, then they will be required to take an additional 30 contact hours. There must also be a signed joint protocol in place with a physician. For specific guidelines, please contact the NJSBN.

A 1992 bill passed which mandates insurance reimbursement for RNs at the same rate as that of physicians. Medicaid pays for NPs and CNSs as well. Medicare reimbursement is also available.

New Mexico

The BRN licenses NPs, CNSs, and RNAs. The Department of Health regulates CNMs. All must be nationally certified as such. There are about 350 of these advanced practice nurses. CNSs with a masters's degree in Nursing and ANCC certification may perform counseling/psychotherapy services. They may not diagnose or prescribe.

All of these nurses may work independently of physicians, but only the CNPs have prescriptive authority, including Schedule II-V drugs. The CNP must have experience with writing prescriptions, have a special license, have a DEA number, and maintain a formulary list.

There is specific legislation since 1987 that assists with third-party reimbursement and these nurses are billing insurance companies. NPs may receive Medicaid reimbursement at the 90% rate of physicians. Some Medicare reimbursement is also allowed in rural areas and in long-term care facilities. The BRN says that the only barrier for CNSs to practice in New Mexico is the MSN requirement.

New York

Nurse Practitioners in 12 subspecialties are recognized by the BRN. There are 34 NPs in psychiatry. Counseling is under the definition of practice for nurses. The only restriction of title is that nurses may not describe themselves or what they do using the terms "psychologist" or "psychological."

Certification as an NP requires completion of a program registered by New York which prepares NPs *or* certification by a national certifying body as an NP that is acceptable by the BRN. The only program for psychiatric NPs listed with the BRN is the State University of New York (SUNY) at Stonybrook. CNSs and CRNAs are not recognized at all.

Psychiatric NPs may work in independent settings, but must have a collaborative relationship and practice protocols with a physician. This need not be a supervisory relationship.

Prescriptive privileges (including Schedule II-IV) are available after the NP has completed a course on pharmacotherapeutics and one on New York and federal laws regarding prescriptions and record keeping. They may have individual DEA numbers. Although NPs may prescribe independently, they still need to have a collaborative relationship with a physician in place. CNMs may also prescribe (limited to their specialty).

NPs are able to bill for third-party reimbursement; there is no specific legislation that assists with this. NPs may bill for Medicaid and receive reimbursement at the same rate as doctors. Medicare reimburses at 85% of physicians' fees in rural areas. The main barrier to practice here is that only NPs are recognized as advanced practice nurses. For specific regulations regarding NP certification, please contact the BRN for their "Certification of NPs" booklet that contains all information and application materials.

North Carolina

There are about 628 APNs in North Carolina. NPs are regulated and defined under Title 21 of the North Carolina Administrative Code, Chapter 36. Other APNs are able to practice via an interpretive statement and general recognition of nurses performing advanced skills (see G. S. 90-171.43 (B) and Rule .0223). They include CRNAs and CNMs. No regulations define CNSs at present.

The PMHN may perform "psychotherapy" which is considered an advanced nursing intervention and falls within the scope of nursing practice (see statement from BRN on this). The PMHN needs to have a master's degree in nursing directly related to mental health, but ANCC certification is not required. PMHNs may work independently of physicians, but need to have a supervisory physician who is available for emergencies (who doesn't have to be on-site). The same is true for NPs.

Only NPs have prescriptive privileges (using written standard protocols that include schedules 2, 2N, 3, 3N, 4, and 5). Physician supervision is required. (For prescriptive privilege parameters, see .0008-9 of Chapter 36.) They must obtain a DEA number.

For insurance reimbursement though, the PMHN must be ANCC certified. Specific legislation passed on October 1, 1993 that assists with nurse reimbursement. PMHNs use the term "RN," just like all others in the state. Medicaid reimburses the same as that of physicians. Medicare reimburses in rural areas and in skilled nursing homes. Champus will pay as well. These APNs experience some difficulty despite the legislation (see 21 NAC 36.0223 [A]). The main barrier has been reimbursement, but not as much since the passage of the new law. The BRN would like to see clearer and stronger language in the Nursing Practice Act regarding advanced practice/CNSs. The 1996 amendments were a step forward, though. Especially important would be to set specific educational and practice standards for the other types of APNs. The attitude varies as to the role of the APN in North Carolina.

North Dakota

Advanced practice nurses are included in the statute/administrative rules. They include NPs, CNMs, CRNAs, and CNSs. There are currently over 300 such nurses in North Dakota. Psychiatric NPs and CNSs are able to perform counseling/psychotherapy if trained to do so. Educational requirements include a master's degree in nursing directly related to mental health, and they must be ANCC certified. These nurses may work independently of physicians. Since 1995, the BRN requires all APNs to be trained at the master's level before application is made.

They may apply for prescriptive privileges if they have pharmacology coursework (30 hours). They do need to have a written collaborative statement with a physician for their prescriptive privileges. ARNPs may prescribe (Schedule II-V) drugs and obtain their own DEA number.

There are specific laws requiring insurance reimbursement for nurses, and they are legally able to bill third-party payors. Medicaid reimburses FNPs and PNPs at 75% of the rate for doctors. CNMs are reimbursed at a 100% rate. Medicare reimbursement is not a problem and is managed by Blue Cross/Blue Shield. This insurance company reimburses all APNs at 75% of allowable charges.

Managed Care contracts are currently not available, but many APNs are working to help in this area. The main barrier to practice here is the few numbers of nurses to make their presence known to legislative bodies. There is mixed response among physicians as to advanced practice in general.

Ohio

Until 1997, the only advanced practice currently being recognized in Ohio are those in pilot programs. Effective since 10/1/93, the Proposed Rules Revision of the NPA defines advanced practice nurses as RNs approved by the state. They include an Ohio RN license, completion of a program in advanced nursing, have had at least three years and 3,000 hours as an RN, be certified as an NP, CNS, or CNM, be employed by the following universities (CRNAs are excluded). These rules are proposed for programs at Case Western Reserve University and Wright University only, and not the general population at large. These APN licenses are good until the year 2000. SB154 did pass in 1996 to license all APNs and was signed by the governor in June of 1996.[23] Rules and regulations will then be written by the BRN which will allow for licensing of APNs outside of the university setting.

Their scope of practice will be more limited than those at the university research projects and will exclude prescriptive privileges. The BRN plans to finalize all rules and regulations by the end of 1996 and will implement them as soon as they are completed (expected January 1997).

Some NPs are being paid by insurance companies. MediCaid does not recognize APNs even though mandated by the State Attorney General.

Oklahoma

The NPA defines advanced practitioners to include: ARNPs, CNSs, CNMs, and CRNAs. Currently, the BRN recognizes 262 ARNPs and 79 CNSs. Counseling and psychotherapy may be performed if the nurse is educated for this. There are many certifying boards recognized by the BRN, including the ANCC. This certification is not mandatory for the CNS. NPs must be formally trained and certified as such.

ARNPs may work independently of physicians, but do not have prescriptive authority. A bill was introduced in 1994 that asked for prescriptive privileges without physician supervision, but was amended to allow for physician supervision for Schedule III-V drugs only.

There are no specific laws in place to assist with reimbursement at this time. FNPs and PNPs are the only ARNPs currently receiving any Medicaid reimbursement at the 85% rate of doctor's fees. Medicare is not available.

Oregon

NPs and CNMs are certified by the BRN. CRNAs and CNSs are not officially recognized, but can practice anyway. The BRN is looking into options to include them. They may also bill directly for their services, but with some difficulty. Most advanced practice nurses practice as NPs, including Psychiatric NPs and must be certified as such by the BRN. RNs with master's degrees in counseling are providing counseling and psychotherapy and can do so in private practice, but cannot use the term "NP." There are a total of 870 NPs in Oregon; 144 of these are PMHNs. Only this latter group may perform psychotherapy. To be considered a psychiatric nurse practitioner, you must have graduated from a nurse practitioner program, and have a master's degree in nursing directly related to mental health that prepared you for an advanced role. ANCC certification used to be required, but it is no longer.

The psychiatric mental health nurse practitioner may work independently of physicians and may qualify for prescriptive privileges. All NPs can prescribe via formulary (Schedule III-V) drugs independent of physicians and they also qualify for their own DEA numbers.

Through legal mandates, they are being reimbursed well for their services by insurance companies and they qualify for hospital privileges. Medicaid reimburses NPs the same as they do doctors.

Pennsylvania

APNs are not licensed or certified here, although CNPs may function under an expanded role. They must perform all services under physician supervision. They may perform counseling services. There are no protected titles. No educational or practice requirements are spelled out for the PMHN. The BRN says they have no PMHNs. CNMs practice under protocols and collaboration with a physician.

Prescriptive privileges will be available under physician supervision and include controlled substances (III-V). The Rules and Regulations have not yet been approved so it has not gone into effect yet. They may also apply for their own DEA number.

There are no laws governing reimbursement, and nurses are not listed on managed care contracts. CRNAs, CRNPs, and Certified CNSs are able to bill, though. Medicaid reimburses CNPs at the same rate as that of physicians. Advanced practice for nurses seems to be very marginal.

Rhode Island

NPs, CNSs, CNMs, and CRNAs are recognized here. The last group has just begun the process of defining rules and regulations. There are no practice requirements for physician collaboration or supervision.

Yet NPs and CNMs who have prescriptive privileges must do so under physician supervision. The list of formulary medications includes controlled substances (Schedule IV-V). The NP must complete 30 hours of pharmacology prior to application and must complete 30 hours of continuing education every six years. CNMs can apply for DEA numbers, but not NPs as of yet. This will most likely change soon.

In June of 1990, there was legislation that passed to mandate reimbursement for psychiatric CNSs and CNMs. In January 1992, legislation passed that allows for independent reimbursement of NPs and Psychiatric CNSs to receive funding from health centers funded by the Department of Health. Medicaid reimbursement has been established legally, but the fees have not been set and implemented. In 1995 legislation was passed that allows for CNPs and psychiatric CNSs to be reimbursed if in collaboration or employed by a physician. The state is also considering giving CNSs prescriptive privileges.

South Carolina

Advanced practice nurses are officially recognized in this state. Currently, there are 275 NPs, 80 CNMs, and 27 CNSs. They are allowed to work independently without physician supervision and provide counseling and psychotherapy services, except when operating under an expanded role and doing "medical acts." Then, he or she must have physician support, collaboration, and must follow written protocols. NPs and clinical nurse specialists functioning in an expanded role are covered in Article 2, Section 91-6 of the Nurse Practice Act. These nurses must be nationally certified as such, that is, NP, CNS, and so forth. Nurse midwives are considered NPs. Since January 1, 1995, all new ARNP nurses are required to hold a master's degree in nursing in their related area as well as national certification. Currently, there is no special licensure or certification by the BRN, but national certification deems the nurse "certified."

Prescriptive privileges are available under physician directed protocols. Only NPs and CNSs may prescribe Schedule V drugs. DEA numbers are available.

There are no legislative measures to assist in third-party billing, but ARNPs are able to bill insurance companies. The titles NP and CNS are defined in the Nurse Practice Act for use in Medicaid (80% of physicians' rates) and Medicare reimbursement. The SBRN says that physicians and other mental health providers have a positive attitude toward ARNPs in this state.

South Dakota

The South Dakota BRN recognizes CRNAs, CNMs, and CNPs under the Nurse Practice Act, Chapters 20:48, 20:62, 36-99, and 36-9A. Since July

1, 1995 they also recognize clinical nurse specialists. These ARNPs must be under the supervision of a doctor and can perform "delegated medical functions" under the physician's guidance. There is no restriction on the use of the terms counseling and psychotherapy, but the nurse must have the necessary credentials to perform these roles. Board certification (BRN) is necessary for NPs and NMs. These titles are also defined and protected within the Nurse Practice Act. Counseling is considered under the Nurse Practice Act for RNs. NPs and CNMs must be certified nationally and by the BRN. CNSs must have a MSN degree and national certification.

Prescriptive privileges are available for CNPs and CNMs, but only under physician supervision. Schedule III-V drugs may be prescribed and DEA numbers are available. The ARNPs may bill for third-party payment, but it is usually done under the supervising physician.

Since 1980, special legislation has existed to help with third-party reimbursement. NPs and CNMs receive Medicaid reimbursement at 90% of physician's fees. CNPs are defined for use in Medicare reimbursement. Up-to-date information about reimbursement issues can be obtained by calling the Division of Insurance at (605) 773-3563, and the Department of Social Services at (605) 773-3495. Barriers to advanced practice are: physician dependent practice, and exclusionary language of private insurance contracts.

Tennessee

RNs may expand their role as long as they are competent, by education and experience, to do so. Although the four types of APNs are able to practice as such, there is no official recognition by the BRN.

NPs and CNSs (who qualify as an APN) may obtain prescriptive privileges for noncontrolled substances only. To obtain prescriptive privileges they must have a Certificate of Fitness issued by the BRN. In order for this, they must have a master's degree in a nursing specialty and be nationally certified, and have three quarter-hours of pharmacology training. The site of practice must have prior approval as well, and the nurse must have a supervisory physician to prescribe. The Tennessee Nurses Association is trying to introduce legislation that will eliminate the need for site approval.

All of the APNs can receive Medicaid reimbursement (now called Tenn Care) at a rate of 90% of physician's fees. All of the APNs may receive Medicare reimbursement. A 1994 law assists with reimbursement to CNMs. CRNAs, NPs, and psychiatric CNSs have negotiated private insurer reimbursement. House Bill (90-3) was introduced in 1995 and is being considered by the Senate to mandate reimbursement.

Texas

Through a credentialing process (not licensure) established by Rule 221, advanced practice nurses are recognized in Texas. These advanced nurse practitioners include nurse midwives, nurse practitioners, nurse anesthetists, and clinical nurse specialists. Clinical specialists in psychiatric mental-health nursing are able to perform counseling and psychotherapy services and the title is protected by the Administrative rules. CNSs must have a master's degree in nursing in an area related to mental health, *or* have a master's degree in nursing and be certified by ANCC as a clinical specialist in psychiatric mental health (adult or child). A nurse with a master's degree in a related field, for example, counseling or psychology, may petition the BRN if they are ANCC certified and meet the other requirements. Other than this last group, certification is not mandated.

Psychiatric CNSs may work independently of doctors only if they do not manage medical aspects of care, such as prescribing drugs. In that case, all APNs must have a collaborative relationship with a physician and use established protocols. In order for these nurses to have prescriptive authority they must demonstrate evidence of pharmacotherapeutics education at the graduate level. Legislation passed in 1995 that allows for prescriptive authority for ANPs regardless of site and includes legend drugs only.

CNSs may bill for third-party payment. The Insurance Code SB 2055 was passed in September 1993, and provides for small businesses to reimburse these specialists (it became effective January 1994). Medicaid reimbursement is available at 85% of physician's fees. There is a law that seeks to prohibit discrimination against various health care providers, but nurses have not been listed here yet. The present barriers to practice for PMHNs are reimbursement issues as just stated, a need for broader prescriptive privileges, and lack of clinical (in-patient) privileges.

Utah

In Title 58, Chapter 31:13, the Nurse Practice Act defines advanced practice registered nurses (ARNPs) as nurse practitioners, nurse specialists, and psychiatric mental health specialists. Utah also recognizes nurse anesthetists. If these ARNPs have applicable knowledge and education, they may perform counseling. Only the PMHN specialist may perform and use the term psychotherapy. The Utah Rules of the Board of Nursing defines psychotherapy in R156-31-3(j). Educational requirements include a master's degree in nursing directly related to mental health *and* ANCC certification as a clinical nurse specialist. All ARNPs regardless of specialty must have their respective national certifications.

These nurses may work independently of a physician except when they have prescriptive authority. In this case, a written consultation and referral plan must be submitted at the time of application. APNs may prescribe Schedule III-V drugs and obtain their own DEA number. Educational requirements for prescriptive privileges include 30 hours of the following: advanced health assessment, pharmacology, and psychopharmacology (see R156-31-8-9).

ARNPs may bill for third-party payment, but experience closed managed care panels despite some antidiscrimination language in the laws. Some payors refuse to acknowledge and reimburse nonphysician providers. There is no law regarding third-party reimbursement, but legislation has been proposed this year to add ARNPs to the state's evidence code. Medicaid has been paying FNPs and PNPs the same as that of doctors. Medicare is also available. The reimbursement issue seems to be the main barrier to practice, but there is also the attitude by physicians that ARNPs are undereducated. Many doctors do improve their support after developing relationships with ARNPs.

Vermont

Vermont endorses (licenses) 265 advanced practice registered nurses as NPs, Psychiatric CNSs, CNMs, and CRNAs. Of these, about 95%–98% are in private practice with physicians. The BRN is considering allowing non-psych CNSs to be added to the list of APNs. Psychiatric CNSs may perform counseling/psychotherapy services and must be ANCC certified.

They may work independently of physician supervision if they do not hold prescriptive privileges; in this case, they must have a collaborative relationship with a doctor and have established mutual protocols. APNs may prescribe Schedule II-V drugs and obtain a DEA number.

Most nurses do not seem to be billing for third-party payment, but are able to do so. I suspect that if they are in practice with physicians they are billing directly under the doctor. Blue Cross/Blue Shield reimburses Psychiatric NPs. FNPs, PNPs, and CNMs receive Medicaid reimbursement the same as doctors. Although no specific legislation exists to assist with reimbursement, APNs are increasingly being paid.

Virginia

Advanced practice nurses are recognized here. Clinical nurse specialists must be registered with the BRN; there are 327 of these (unknown how many are psychiatric). The other types of nurses (NPs, CRNAs, and CNMs) are all licensed (total is 2,276). There is no category for psychiatric NP. The psychiatric CNS may perform counseling/psychotherapy based upon education. They must have a master's degree in nursing or a related field and some form of national certification (BRN not allowed to limit type).

These CNSs may work independently of physicians, unless they have prescriptive authority. In this case, they must qualify as an APN and have a written practice agreement with a physician. The same is true of NPs and CNMs. CRNAs are excluded from prescribing.

Virginia Acts of Assembly—Chapter 7 (38.2-4221)—states that CNSs must be paid for mental health services performed. The other types of APNs may bill, but do not always get paid. Medicaid pays at 100% of physician payment. MediCare is excluded.

Washington

In Washington, you must be licensed as a registered nurse and have graduated from a nurse practitioner program, and/or be an ANCC certified psychiatric mental-health clinical nurse specialist. The education must be either a master's in nursing or one in a related field such as counseling. Since January 1995, the master's degree must be in nursing directly related to mental-health. They use the term Advanced Practice Registered Nurse Practitioner (ANRP) for both NPs and CNSs. Accordingly, in Washington state, there is no distinction between them.

They may work independently of physicians and are also able to have prescriptive authority. DEA numbers are available and they may prescribe Schedule V drugs only. Thirty hours of pharmaco therapeutics are needed. Legislation is pending to expand to Schedule II-IV drugs. CRNAs and CNMs are officially recognized here and are also considered ARNPs.

Antidiscrimination laws exist to assist ARNPs to be reimbursed. ARNPs are paid by MedCaid at the 100% rate. MediCare is reimbursed via federal guidelines.

West Virginia

The BRN recognizes APNs as NPs, CNMs, CRNAs, and CNSs. All need to be nationally certified and in 1999, must be master's prepared. Psychiatric CNS's may use the term ''nurse-counselor,'' but not ''counselor'' by itself because there is a separate Board for Licensed Counselors in this state. They must have a master's degree in nursing directly related to mental health and must be ANCC certified as CNSs. They specifically can use the term Clinical Specialist Advanced Practice.

They may work independently of physicians, but must have a collaborative relationship with a doctor if they utilize prescriptive privileges. All APNs may prescribe Schedule III-V drugs and obtain their own DEA number. Malpractice insurance is mandated by the BRN. Also, they must have pharmacology education and have written guidelines/protocols with a physician.

APNs may bill for third-party payment, but are doing so with some difficulty. Legislation was passed in 1983, but no rules have been written from it to help with this more specifically. Medicaid and Medicare reimbursement have been accounted for by Legislative Rule 19CSR7, with variable results. One main barrier beside the reimbursement issue has been concerned legislators who have restricted prescriptive authority for psychoactive drugs. Generally, though, the attitude is positive for advanced practice here.

Wisconsin

Under Chapter N 8, the BRN recognizes APNs as those nurses who are nationally certified as NPs, CNMs, CRNAs, and CNSs. After July 1, 1998, applicants must have a master's in nursing or a related health field. Psychiatric NPs and CNSs may practice psychotherapy/counseling if trained to do so

All APNs may be issued a "certificate" to prescribe. To qualify, they must have at least 45 contact hours in clinical pharmacology/therapeutics within three years of the application, and have passed an examination by the BRN. Continuing education requirements are at least eight contact hours per year in pharmacology relevant to the specialty area. Independent prescriptive authority includes Schedule II-V drugs, but the APN must facilitate collaboration with two health care providers, one of which must be a physician. This does not mean supervision. DEA numbers are available, and the BRN mandates malpractice insurance.

MediCaid reimbursement is available to all master's prepared APNs if nationally certified. MediCare is per the federal guidelines. Third-party reimbursement legislation will be introduced by the Wisconsin Nurses Association in 1997. To assist with their efforts, please call the WNA at (608) 221-0383. The lack of reimbursement is the biggest barrier to practice.

Wyoming

The BRN says they only have two advanced practitioners of nursing listed. APNs are defined to include nurse midwives, nurse practitioners, clinical specialists, and certified nurse anesthetists. Educationally, these ANPs must be trained in a program that prepares for advanced practice *and* be nationally certified in their specialty. Psychiatric specialists may perform counseling services if in collaboration with a physician. Even though they may not work independently, they do not require direct supervision.

Prescriptive privileges are available in Wyoming after the APN has completed 30 contact hours of education in pharmacology within the five-year period before the date of application. Along with this is the requirement that the APN must have completed 400 hours of practice within the two years preceding the application, *and* submit signed copies of current collaborative practice plans. Privileges include Schedule III-V drugs. They may apply for their own DEA number. The BRN mandates malpractice insurance for them as well. Even without prescriptive privileges, the APN must submit at the time of application, a written plan specifying the collaborative relationship with a physician or other appropriate health care provider, including referral of clients. Under Chapter 4 of the Nurse Practice Act, 60 hours of continuing education and 400 hours of experience are required for renewal biennially, *or* maintain national certification plus 30 hours of continuing education. There are anti-discrimination laws regrading third-party reimbursement. MediCaid is available at the 100% rate. MediCare is excluded.

NOTES

1. Pearson, L. (Ed.). (1996, January). Annual Update of how each state stands on legislative issues affecting advanced nursing practice. *The Nurse Practitioner*, 10–70.
2. American Psychiatric Nurses Association. (1996, July). Prescriptive authority chart. Congress on Advanced Practice in Psychiatric Nursing, 1–8.
3. Carson, W. (1996, February). Prescriptive authority chart. American Nurses Association Nurse Practice Counsel, 1–8.
4. Ibid.
5. Ibid.
6. Huff, B. (Ed.). (1996). *Physician's Desk Reference.* Oradell, NJ: Litton Industries, 2687.
7. Lepler, M. (September 2, 1996). Managed care brings APNs mixed blessings (Part 1). *NURSEweek, 1,* 22–23.
8. Lepler, M. (September 16, 1996). Managed care brings APNs mixed blessings (Part 2). *NURSEweek, 1,* 22.

9. California Board of Registered Nursing. (July 8, 1994). *Clinical Nurse Specialist Task Force Memo.*

10. California State Board of Nursing. (1988). *Nursing Practice Act with rules and regulations.* Sacramento, CA: CBRN.

11. *NURSEweek.* (1996, August). Legislative bulletin. *NURSEweek*, 6.

12. *NURSEweek* (Sept. 16, 1996). Legislative Bulletin, *NURSEweek, 19* (19), 7.

13. CBRN, 62–66.

14. American Nurses Association. *Code for nurses.* Washington, DC: Author.

15. American Nurses Association. (1996, July/August). In brief. *American Nurse*, 6.

16. Pearson, L. (Ed.). (1994, January). Annual update of how each state stands on legislative issues affecting advanced nursing practice. *The Nurse Practitioner*, 26.

17. American Nurses Association. (1994, March). *American Nurse*, 14.

18. Maine State Board of Nursing. (1993). Rules and regulations of the State Board of Nursing. Augusta, ME: Author.

19. Ibid.

20. Maryland Department of Health and Mental Hygiene, 10. 27.12.05). Board of Registered Nursing, 1592-32.

21. American Nurses Association. (1996, September). In brief. *American Nurse 28* (6), 14.

22. American Nurses Association. (1994, July/August). NJSNA leads the way for MSN requirement. *American Nurse*, 14.

23. American Nurses Association. (1996, July/August). In brief. *American Nurse*, 6.

RECOMMENDED JOURNALS, PERIODICALS, AND ANA PUBLICATIONS

The following resources are some important sources of information for you. It will be very useful to you to subscribe to some of the following journals. It is also advisable that you write your own State Board of Nursing and State Nurses Association for essentials that pertain to your scope of practice within your specialty.

JOURNALS/PERIODICALS

American Journal of Nursing (Boulder, CO: American Journal of Nursing Corporation, 12 times/year).

American Journal of Orthopsychiatry (Albany, NY: American Orthopsychiatry Association, 4 times/year).

American Journal of Psychiatry (Washington, DC: American Psychiatric Association, 12 times/year).

American Nurse (Washington: American Nurses Association, 10 times/year).

American Nurses Association Council Perspectives (Washington: ANA: 2–4 times/yr).

Archives of Psychiatric Nursing (Philadelphia, PA: W.B. Saunders, 6 times/year).

Attention Nurses (Glendale: AN, 6 times/year).

California Nurse (San Francisco: California Nurses Association, 10 times/year).

The California Therapist (San Diego: California Association of Marriage and Family Therapists, 6 times/year).

Capitol Update (Washington: ANA, 24 times/year).

Clinical Nurse Specialist: Journal for Advanced Nursing Practice (Rowland Heights, CA: Williams and Wilkins, 6 times/year).

Directory of Psychiatric-Mental Health Nurses in California (San Francisco: CNA, 2nd ed., 1990).

Family Therapy News (Washington: American Association for Marriage and Family Therapy, 6 times/year).

Journal of Marital and Family Therapy (Washington: American Association for Marriage and Family Therapy, 3 times/year).

Journal of Neuropsychology (Bethesda, MD: American Psychological Society, 6 times/year).

Journal of Neuroscience Nursing (Chicago, IL: Association of Neuroscience Nursing, 6 times/year).

Journal of Nursing Educators (Thorofare, NJ: SLACK, Inc., 9 times/year).

Journal of Pediatric Psychology (New York, NY: Plenum Press, 6 times/year).

Journal of the American Psychiatric Nurses Association (St. Louis: Mosby YearBook, Inc., 6 times/year).

National Directory of Nurse Practition Programs (Washington, DC: National Organization of Nurse Practitioner Faculties, 1996). (A Directory).

Nurse Practitioner: The American Journal of Primary Health Care (Washington, DC: National Association of Nurse Practitioners, 6 times/year).

Nurses in Advanced Practice (Seattle: Washington State Nurses Association, 1990). (A Directory).

Nurses Resources (Washington: ANA, 1993).

Nurseweek (Sunnyvale: Nurseweek, 52 times/year). (For a complete guide to national nursing organizations, please see January 17, 1994 issue.)

Nursing Trends & Issues (Washington, DC: American Nurses Association, 12 times/year).

Psychiatric Services (Washington, DC: American Psychiatric Association, 12 times/year).

Psychiatry: Interpersonal and Biological Processes (New York, NY: Guilford Press, 6 times/year).

Psychopharmacology Bulletin (Rockville, MD: National Institutes of Health, 3–4 times/year).

Psychotherapy Quarterly (Utica, NY:; American Psychological Association, 4 times/year).

RN Times (LA: *Los Angeles Times*, 12 times/year).

AMERICAN NURSES ASSOCIATION PUBLICATIONS

Code for Nurses With Interpretive Statements, 1985.

Directory of Certification Examination Review Courses, 1996.

How to Take ANCC Certification Examinations, 1994.

National Directory of ANCC-Certified Nurses in Advanced Practice, 1995.

Nurse Entrepreneur: A Reference Manual for Business Design, 1989.

Nursing: A Social Policy Statement, 1987.

Psychiatric and Mental Health Clinical Nurse Specialists: Distribution and Utilization, 1986.

Reimbursement Manual: How to Get Paid for Your Advanced Practice Nursing Services, 1993.

The Role of the Clinical Nurse Specialist, 1986.

Self-Employment in Nursing: The Basics of Starting a Business, 1993

Scope and Standards of Advanced Practice Registered Nursing, 1996.

Scope and Standards of Addictions Nursing Practice, 1997.

Standards of Child and Adolescent Psychiatric and Mental Health Nursing Practice, 1985.

Standards of Psychiatric-Consultation Liaison Nursing Practice, 1990.

Standards of Psychiatric and Mental Health Nursing Practice, 1982, 1994.

Statement on Psychiatric and Mental Health Nursing, 1976.

STATE BOARDS OF NURSING AND NURSING ORGANIZATIONS

STATE BOARDS OF NURSING

Alabama BN
RSA Plaza, Suite 250
770 Washington Ave.
Montgomerey, AL 36130
(205) 242-4060

Alaska Board of Nursing Licensing
Department of Commerce and
  Economic Development
Division of Occupational
  Licensing
P.O. Box 110806
Juneau, AK 99811
(907) 464-2544

Arizona BN
2001 West Camelback Rd.,
Suite 350
Phoenix, AZ 85015
(602) 255-5092

Arkansas SBN
University Tower Bldg.

1123 South University Ave.,
Suite 800
Little Rock, AR 72204
(501) 686-2700

California BRN
P.O. Box 944210
400 R St., Suite 4030
Sacramento, CA 95814
(916) 322-3350

Colorado BN
1650 Braodway, Suite 670
Denver, CO 80202
(303) 894-2430

Connecticut Board of Examiners
  for Nursing
Department of Health Services
150 Washington St.
Hartford, CT 06106
(203) 566-1041

Delaware BN
Margaret O'Neill Bldg.
Federal and Court Streets
P.O. Box 1401
Dover, DE 19903
(302) 739-4522

District of Columbia BN
Department of Consumer and
  Regulatory Affairs
614 H St., N.W., Room 904
P.O. Box 37200
Washington, DC 20001
(202) 727-7461

Florida SBN
111 East Coastline Dr., Suite 516
Jacksonville, FL 32202
(904) 359-6331

Georgia BN, RN
166 Pryor St., S.W., Suite 400
Atlanta, GA 30303
(404) 656-3943

Hawaii SBN
P.O. Box 3469
Honolulu, HI 96801
(808) 548-3086

Idaho BN
280 North 8th St., Suite 210
Boise, ID 83720
(208) 334-3110

Illinois Department of
  Professional Regulation
320 West Washington St.,
  3rd Floor
Springfield, IL 62786
(217) 785-0800

Indiana SBN
Health Professions Service Bureau
402 West Washington St.,

Room 041
Indianapolis, IN 46204
(317) 232-2960

Iowa BN
1223 East Court
Des Moines, IA 50319
(515) 281-3255

Kansas BN
Landon State Office Building
900 S.W. Jackson, Room 551
Topeka, KS 66612
(913) 296-4929

Kentucky SBN
312 Whittington Parkway,
  Suite 300
Louisville, KY 40222
(502) 329-7000

Louisiana SBN
150 Baronne St., Room 912
New Orleans, LA 70112
(504) 568-5464

Maine SBN
State House Station
P.O. Box 158
Augusta, ME 04433
(207) 624-5275

Maryland BN
Metro Executive Center
4201 Patterson Ave.
Baltimore, MD 21215
(410) 764-4747

Massachusetts BRN
100 Cambridge St., Suite 1519
Boston, MA 02202
(617) 727-9961

Michigan BN
P.O. Box 30018
Lansing, MI 48909
(517) 373-1600

Minnesota BN
2700 University Ave. West,
Suite 108
St. Paul, MN 55114
(612)642-0567

Mississippi BN
239 North Lamar, Suite 401
Jackson, MS 39201
(601) 359-6170

Missouri SBN
3605 Missouri Blvd.
P.O. Box 656
Jefferson City, MO 65102
(314) 751-0681

Montana SBN
Department of Commerce
Arcade Bldg., Lower Level
111 North Jackson
P.O. Box 200513
Helena, MT 59620
(406) 444-4279

Nebraska BN
State House Station
P.O. Box 95007
Lincoln, NE 68509
(402) 471-2115

Nevada SBN
1281 Terminal Way, Suite 116
Reno, NV 89502
(702) 786-2778

New Hampshire BN
Division of Public Health Services
Health and Welfare Building
#6 Hazen Dr.

Concord, NH 03301
(603) 271-2323

New Jersey BN
124 Halsey St., 6th Floor
P.O. Box 45010
Newark, NJ 07101
(201) 504-6493

New Mexico BN
4253 Montgomerey N.E., Suite 130
Albuquerque, NM 87109
(505) 841-8340

New York SBN
State Education Department
Cultural Education Center
Albany, NY 12230
(518) 474-3843

North Carolina BN
P.O. Box 2129
Raleigh, NC 27602
(919) 782-3211

North Dakota BN
919 South 7th St., Suite 504
Bismarck, ND 58504
(701) 224-2974

Ohio BN
77 South High St., 17th Floor
Columbus, OH 43266
(614) 466-3847

Oklahoma Board of Registration
   and Nursing Education
2915 North Classen Blvd.,
   Suite 524
Oklahoma City, OK 73106
(405) 525-2076

Oregon SBN
800 NE Oregon St. #25
Portland, OR 97232
(503) 731-4745

Pennsylvania SBN
P.O. Box 2649
Harrisburg, PA 17105
(717) 783-7142

Rhode Island Board of Nursing
   Registration and Nursing
   Education
Cannon Health Building,
   Room 104
#3 Capitol Hill
Providence, RI 02908
(401) 277-2827

South Carolina SBN
220 Executive Center Dr.,
Suite 220
Columbia, SC 29210
(803) 731-1648

South Dakota BN
3307 South Lincoln Ave.
Sioux Falls, SD 57105
(605) 335-4973

Tennessee SBN
283 Plus Park Blvd.
Nashville, TN 37427
(615) 367-6232

Texas Board of Nurse Examiners
9109 Burnet Rd., Suite 104
P.O. Box 140466
Austin, TX 78714
(512) 835-4880

Utah SBN
Divison of Occupational and Pro-
fessional Licensing
Heber M. Wells Building, 4th Floor
160 East 300 St.
P.O. Box 45802
Salt Lake City, UT 84145
(801) 530-6628

Vermont SBN
109 State St.
Montpelier, VT 05609
(802) 828-2396

Virginia SBN
6606 West Broad St., Fourth Floor
Richmond, VA 23230
(804) 662-9909

Washington SBN
Division of Professional Licensing
P.O. Box 47864
Olympia, WA 98504
(206) 453-2686

West Virginia Board of Examiners
   for Registered Nurses
101 Dee Drive
Charleston, WV 25311
(304) 558-3692

Wisconsin BN
Room 174, P.O. Box 8935
Madison, WI 53708
(608) 266-0145

Wyoming SBN
Garrett Building, 2nd Fl.
2301 Central Ave.
Cheyenne, WY 82002
(307) 777-7601

Nursing Associations/ Organizations

National:

Addictions Nursing
CARN Certification
National League of Nursing
350 Hudson St.
New York, NY 10009

Advocates for Child Psychiatric
  Nursing
1211 Locust St.
Philadelphia, PA 19107
(215) 545-2843

American Academy of Nurse
  Practitioners
Capitol Station, LBJ Building
Austin, TX 78711
(512) 442-4262

American College of Nurse
  Midwives
Directory of NM Programs
1522 K St. N.W., Suite 1000
Washington, DC 20005
(202) 289-0171

American Nurses Association
600 Maryland Ave. Suite 100W
Washington, DC 20024
(800) 274-4ANA
(202) 554-4444

American Psychiatric Nurses
  Association
1200 19th St. NW, Suite 300
Washington, DC 20036-2422
(202) 857-1133

Drug and Alcohol Nursing
  Association
660 Lonely Cottage Dr.
Upper Black Eddy, PA 18972
(610) 847-5396

National Alliance of Nurse
  Practitioners
325 Pennsylvania Ave., S.E.
Washington, DC 20003
(202) 675-6350

National Association of Neonatal
  Nurses
Directory of NNP Programs

1304 Southpoint Blvd., Suite 280
Petaluma, CA 94954
(800) 451-3795

State:

Alabama State Nurses Association
360 North Hull St.
Montgomery, AL 36104
(205) 262-8321

Alaska Nurses Association
237 East Third Ave.
Anchorage, AK 99501
(907) 274-0827

Arizona Nurses Association
1850 East Southern Ave., Suite 1
Tempe, AZ 85282
(602) 831-0404

Arkansas Nurses Association
117 South Cedar St.
Little Rock, AR
(501) 664-5853

California Alliance of
  Advanced Practice Nurses
  (CAAPN)
9852 Katella Ave., Suite 407
Anaheim, CA 92804
(714) 772-3332

California Association of
  Psychiatric Mental Health
  Nurses in Advanced Practice
12021 Wilshire Blvd., Suite 797
Los Angeles, CA 90025
(310) 364-0960

California Nurses Association
  (not a part of ANA)
1145 Market St., Suite 1100
San Francisco, CA 94103
(415) 864-4141

California Nurses Association/
    ANA
P.O. Box 225
3010 Wilshire Blvd.
Los Angeles, CA 90010
(800) 646-4262

Colorado Nurses Association
5453 East Evans Place
Denver, CO 80222
(303) 757-7483

Connecticut Nurses Association
Meritech Business Park
377 Research Parkway, Suite 2D
Meriden, CT 06450
(203) 238-3437

Delaware Nurses Association
2634 Capitol Trail, Suite A
Newark, DE 19711
(302) 368-2333

District of Columbia Nurses
    Association
5100 Wisconsin Ave., N.W.,
Suite 306
Washington, DC 20016
(202) 244-2705

Florida Nurses Association
P.O. Box 536985
Orlando, FL 32853
(407) 896-3261

Georgia Nurses Association
1362 West Peachtree St., N.W.
Atlanta, GA 30339
(404) 876-4624

Hawaii Nurses Association
677 Ala Moana Blvd., Suite 301
Honolulu, HI 96813
(808) 521-8361

Idaho Nurses Association
200 North Fourth St., Suite 20
Boise, ID 83702
(208) 345-1163

Illinois Nurses Association
300 South Wacker Dr., Suite 2200
Chicago, IL 60606
(312) 360-2300

Indiana State Nurses Association
2915 North High School Rd.
Indianapolis, IN 46224
(317) 299-4575

Iowa Nurses Association
1501 42nd St., Suite 471
West Des Moines, IA 50266
(515) 255-0495

Kansas State Nurses Association
700 S.W. Jackson, Suite 601
Topeka, KS 66603
(913) 233-8638

Kentucky Nurses Association
1400 South First St.
P.O. Box 2616
Louisville, KY 40201
(502) 637-8236

Louisiana State Nurses Association
712 Transcontinental Dr.
Metairie, LA 70001
(504) 889-1030

Maine State Nurses Association
P.O. Box 2240
Augusta, ME 04330
(207) 622-1057

Maryland Nurses Association
849 International Dr.
Airport Square 21, Suite 255
Linthicum, MD 21090
(410) 859-3000

Massachusetts Nurses Association
340 Turnpike St.
Canton, MA 02021
(617) 821-4625

Michigan Nurses Association
2310 Jolly Oak Rd.
Okemos, MI 48864
(517) 349-5818

Minnesota Nurses Association
1295 Bandana Blvd. North,
  Suite 140
St. Paul, MN 55108
(612) 646-4807

Mississippi Nurses Association
135 Bounds St., Suite 100
Jackson, MS 39206
(601) 982-9182

Missouri Nurses Association
206 East Dunklin St., Box 325
Jefferson City, MO 65101
(314) 636-4623

Montana Nurses Association
104 Broadway, Suite G-2
P.O. Box 5718
Helena, MT 59601
(406) 442-6738

Nebraska Nurses Association
941 O St., Suite 707-711
Lincoln, NE 68508
(402) 475-3961

Nevada Nurses Association
3660 Baker Lane, Suite 104
Reno, NV 89509
(702) 825-3555

New Hampshire Nurses
  Association
48 West St.
Concord, NH 03301
(603) 225-3783

New Jersey State Nurses
  Association
320 West State St.
Trenton, NJ 08618
(609) 392-4884/2031

New Mexico Nurses Association
909 Virginia N.E., Suite 101
Albuquerque, NM 87108
(505) 268-7744

New York State Nurses
  Association
2113 Western Ave.
Guilderland, NY 12084
(518) 456-5371

North Carolina Nurses Association
103 Enterprise St., Box 12025
Raleigh, NC 27605
(919) 821-5807

North Dakota Nurses Association
212 North Fourth St.
Bismarck, ND 58501
(701) 223-1385

Ohio Nurses Association
4000 East Main St.
Columbus, OH 43213
(614) 237-5414

Oklahoma Nurses Association
6414 North Sante Fe, Suite A
Oklahoma City, OK 73116
(405) 840-3476

Oregon State Nurses Association
9600 S.W. Oak, Suite 550
Portland, OR 97223
(503) 293-0011

Pennsylvania Nurses Association
2578 Interstate Dr.
P.O. Box 68525
Harrisburg, PA 17106
(717) 657-1222

Rhode Island State Nurses
   Association
300 Ray Dr., Suite 5
Providence, RI 02906
(401) 421-9703

South Carolina Nurses Association
1821 Gadsden St.
Columbia, SC 29201
(803) 252-4781

South Dakota Nurses Association
1505 South Minnesota Ave.,
Suite 6
Sioux Falls, SD 57105
(605) 338-1401

Tennessee Nurses Association
545 Mainstream Dr., Suite 405
Nashville, TN 37228
(615) 254-0350

Texas Nurses Association
7600 Burnet Rd., Suite 440
Austin, TX 78757
(512) 452-0645

Utah Nurses Association
455 East 400 South, Suite 402
Salt Lake City, UT 84111
(801) 322-3439

Vermont Nurses Association
Box 26 Champlain Mill
#1 Main St.

Winooski, VT 05404
(802) 655-7123

Virginia Nurses Association
7113 Three Chpt Rd.
Richmond, VA 23226
(804) 282-1808

Washington State Nurses
   Association
2505 Second Ave., Suite #500
Seattle, WA 98121
(206) 443-9762

West Virginia Nurses Association
101 Dee Dr.
P.O. Box 1946
Charleston, WV 25327
(304) 342-1169

Wisconsin Nurses Association
6117 Monona Dr.
Madison, WI 53716
(608) 221-0383

Wyoming Nurses Association
Majestic Building, Room 305
1603 Capitol Ave.
Cheyenne, WY 82001
(307) 635-3955

Other Resources

Office of the President
The White House
Washington, DC 20500
(202) 456-1414

U.S. House of Representatives
The Capitol
First and Independence S.E.
Washington, DC 20515
(202) 224-3121

U.S. Senate
The Capitol
First and Consitution N.E.
Washington, DC 20510
(202) 224-3121

Health Resources
  and Services Administration
Bureau of Health Professions
Division of Nursing
5600 Fishers Lane, Room 9-35
Rockville, MD 20857
(301) 443-5786

Health Care Financing
  Administration (HCFA)
Security Office Park Bldg.
Room 1A11
7800 Security Blvd.
Baltimore, MD 21207
(410) 597-5110

PSYCHIATRIC MENTAL-HEALTH NURSE PRACTITIONER PROGRAMS

For a listing of CNS programs in Psychiatric Mental-Health Nursing, call the ANA at (800) 274-4ANA. For a complete listing of *all* types of NP programs, contact the National Organization of Nurse Practitioner Faculties to order a directory. Their address is: NONPF, One Dupont Circle, Suite 530, Washington, D.C., 20036, (202) 452-1405. Below is a listing of PMHN NP programs.[1]

PMHN NP PROGRAMS

Arizona State University
College of Nursing
Beth Vaughn-Wrobel, EdD
Tempe, AZ 85287
(602) 965-2653

California State University, Long
  Beach
Department of Nursing
Dr. Colleen Sparks or Ms. Martha
  Siegel
1250 Bellflower Blvd.

Long Beach, CA 90840
(213) 985-4657 or 985-4473

Case Western Reserve University
  (Ohio)
Frances Payne Bolton School of
  Nursing
Donna Hassik
2121 Abington Rd.
Cleveland, OH 44106
(216) 368-2540

Florida International University
School of Nursing – ARNP
  Program
Shirley Belock, RN, EdD, JD
North Miami, FL 33181

Oregon Health Science University
School of Nursing – EJSN
Cathie Burns, RN, PhD, PNP
3181 S.W. Jackson Park Rd.
Portland, OR 97201
(505) 494-7877

Rivier College (New Hampshire)
School of Nursing
Dr. Joan Lewis
420 Main St.
Nashua, NH 03060
(603) 888-1311, x8529

State University of New York,
  Stonybrook
School of Nursing
Ms. Rose Meyers
Health Sciences Center, Level 2
Stonybrook, NY 11794
(516) 444-3200

University of Alabama,
  Birmingham
School of Nursing
UAB Station
Birmingham, AL 35294
(205) 934-4213

University of California,
  San Francisco
School of Nursing
Barbara Burgel, RN, MS
San Francisco, CA 94143
(415) 476-4953

University of Florida
College of Nursing
Jenny Graham, RN, PhD

P.O. Box 100187
Gainesville, FL 32610
(904) 392-3524

University of Medicine and
  Dentistry of New Jersey
Peter Falk, Registrar
UMDNJ – SON
30 Bergen St./ADMC 1-19
Newark, NJ 07107
(201) 982-5447

University of Massachusetts,
  Lowell
Department of Nursing
Sharon George, RN MS, C
One University Ave.
Lowell, MA 02115
(508) 934-4417

University of Pittsburgh
School of Nursing
Shirley Kobert
426 Victoria Bldg.
Pittsburgh, PA 15261
(412) 624-3827

University of South Florida, Tampa
College of Nursing
Dr. Candace Burns
Tampa, FL 33612
(813) 974-2191

University of Tennessee, Knoxville
Graduate College of Nursing
Dr. Mildred Fenske
1200 Volunteer Blvd.
Knoxville, TN 37996
(615) 974-7609

University of Texas, Arlington
School of Nursing
Wanda Thompson, RNC, FNP,
   EdD
411 Campus Dr.
P.O. Box 19407
Arlington, TX 76019
(817) 273-3073

University of Washington
School of Nursing, SM24
Marie Brown, PhD
Seattle, WA 98195
(206) 685-0815

NOTES

1. National Organization of Nurse Practitioner Faculties. *National Directory of Nurse Practitioner Programs* (1996). Washington, DC: Author.

REFERENCES

American Nurses Association. (1982). *Standards of psychiatric and mental health nursing*. Washington, DC: Author.

American Nurses Association. (1985). *Code for nurses*. Kansas City: Author.

American Nurses Association. (July/August 1996). In brief. *American Nurse, 28* (5). Washington, DC: Author, p. 6.

American Nurses Association. (1986). *Psychiatric and mental health clinical nurse specialists*. Kansas City: Author.

American Nurses Association. (1990). *Standards of psychiatric-consultation liaison nursing practice*. Washington, DC: Author.

American Nurses Association and California Nurses Association. (1992, Fall). *Nursing reimbursement: How to get paid for your services*. Long Beach Seminar.

American Nurses Association. (1992, February 1993, March 1994). *American nurse*. Washington, DC: Author.

American Nurses Association. (1993). *Capital update, 11*(20). Washington, DC: Author.

American Nurses Association. (1993). *ANA Council Perspectives, 2* (3). Washington, DC: Author.

American Nurses Association. (1994, July/August). Certification exam requirements change. *American Nurse*. Washington, DC: Author.

American Nurses Association. (1996, July/August). In Brief. *American Nurse, 28* (5). Washington, DC: Author, p. 6.

American Nurses Association. (1994). *Statement on psychiatric mental health nursing practice*. Kansas City: Author.

American Nurses Association. (1994, July/August). NJSNA leads the way for MSN Requirements. *American Nurse*. Washington, DC: Author.

American Association for Marriage and Family Therapy. (1992). *Family therapy news*. Washington, DC: Author.

American Nurses Credentialing Center. (1996). *ANCC certification catalog*. Reprinted by permission. Washington, DC: Author.

American Psychiatric Association. (1987). *Quick reference to the diagnostic criteria from the DSM III-R*. Washington, DC: Author.

American Psychiatric Association. (1994). *Diagnostic and statistical manual of mental disorders: DSM-IV.* Washington, DC: Author.

American Psychiatric Nurses Association. (1994). *APNA News, 6* (3). Washington, DC: Author.

American Psychiatric Nurses Association. (1996, July). Prescriptive authority chart. Congress on Advanced Practice in Psychiatric Nursing. Washington, DC: Author, pp. 1–8.

Aromando, L. (1989). *Mental health and psychiatric nursing.* Springhouse, PA: Springhouse Corp.

Beck, C., Rawlins, R., & Williams, S. (1988). *Mental health-psychiatric nursing.* St. Louis: C. V. Mosby.

California Association of Marriage and Family Therapists. (1992, November/December). *California Therapist.* Letter to the Editor. San Diego: Author.

California Nurses Association. (1992). CNA protests exclusion of RNs from Victims of Crime Program. *California Nurse, II* (6). San Francisco: Author, pp. 8–9.

California Nurses Association. (1989). *Nursing practice in California: Rights, responsibilities, and regulations* (2d ed.). San Francisco: Author.

California State Board of Nursing. (1994). *Clinical nurse specialist task force memo.* Sacramento.

California State Board of Nursing. (1988). *Nursing Practice Act with rules and regulations.* Sacramento: Department of Consumer Affairs.

Carpenito, L. (1992). *Nursing diagnosis: Application to clinical practice* (4th ed.). Philadelphia: J. B. Lippincott Co.

Carson, W. (1996, February). Prescriptive authority chart. American Nurses Association Nurse Practice Counsel. Washington, DC: American Nurses Association, pp. 1–8.

Department of the Treasury: Internal Revenue Service. (1990). *Tax guide for small business,* #334. Washington, DC: Author.

Durham, J., & Hardin, S. (Eds.). (1986). *The nurse psychotherapist in private practice.* New York: Springer Publishing.

Gray, B. B. (1994, August). Clinical nurse specialists to be studied by BRN. *NURSEweek, 7* (17), p. 16.

Haber, J., McMahon, A., Price-Hoskins, P., & Sideleau, B. (1995). *Comprehensive psychiatric nursing.* St. Louis: Mosby.

Hammers, M. (June 21, 1993). Psych nursing, *RN Times.* Los Angeles: LA Times, pp. 6–7.

Health Care Financing Administration. (1992, June). *Medi-Care Bulletin,* #92-3. Chicago: Author.

Health Care Financing Administation. (1992, July). *Medicaid Bureau.* Chicago: Author.

Hollis, J., & Donn, P. (1989). *Psychological report writing: Theory and practice.* Muncie: Accelerated Development.

Huff, B. (Ed.). (1996). *Physician's Desk Reference.* Oradell, NJ: Litton Industries, p. 2687.

Lepler, M. (September 2, 1996). Managed care brings APNs mixed blessings (Part 1). *NURSEweek, 10* (20). Sunnyvale, CA: Nurseweek Corporation, pp. 1, 22–23.

Lepler, M. (September 16, 1996). Managed care brings APNs mixed blessings (Part 2). *NURSEweek, 9* (19). Sunnyvale, CA: Nurseweek Corporation, pp. 1, 22.

Leslie, D. (1988). *Insurance compensation manual.* San Diego: California Association of Marriage and Family Therapists.

Maine State Board of Nursing. (1993). *Rules and regulations of MSBRN.* Augusta, ME: Author.

Maryland Department of Health and Mental Hygiene. (10.27.12.05), *Rules and regulations.* Baltimore, MD: Author.

McGoldrick, M., & Gerson, R. (1985). *Genograms in family assessment.* New York: Norton & Co.

Meehan, J. (1994, January). ANA expresses disappointment over AMA opposition to APN autonomy. *American Nurse, 26* (1), p. 1.

Mortis, K. (1991). *Third-party reimbursement for R.N.s in Washington State.* Seattle: Washington State Nursing Association.

Moss, R. (1993, November/December). Privileging essential to APN autonomy. *American Nurse, 25* (10), p. 7.

National Organization of Nurse Practitioner Faculties. (1996). *National Directory of Nurse Practitioner Programs.* Washington, DC: Author.

NURSEweek. (August 19, 1996). Legislative bulletin. *NURSEweek 9* (17). Sunnyvale, CA: Nurseweek Corporation, p. 6.

NURSEweek. (1994). Resources: Organizations. *NURSEWeek, 7* (2). Sunnyvale, CA: Nurseweek Corporation, pp. 1–8.

Pearson, L. (Ed.). (1996, January). Annual Update of how each state stands on legislative issues affecting advanced nursing practice. *The Nurse Practitioner, 21* (1). Washington, DC: National Association of Nurse Practitioners, pp. 10–20.

Ridgewood Financial Institute. (1992). *Psychotherapy Finances: Managed Care Handbook.* Jupiter, FL: Author.

Sebastian, L. (1991). Third-Party Reimbursement for Nurses in Advanced Practice. *Perspectives in Psychiatric Care, 27,* (4).

State of California Department of Consumer Affairs. (1990). Laws and Regulations Relating to the Practice of Marriage, Family, and Child Counseling. Sacramento, CA: Author.

Stuart, G., & Sundeen, S. (1995). *Principles and practice of psychiatric nursing.* St. Louis: Mosby.

Thompson, A. (1983). *Ethical concerns in psychotherapy and their legal ramifications.* New York: University Press.

Washington Nurses Association. (1990). *Nurses in Advanced Practice.* Seattle: Washington State Nurses Association.

Webb, L., DiClemente, C., Johnstone, E., Sanders, J., & Perley, R. (Eds.). (1981). *DSM III Training Guide.* New York: Bruner/Mazel.

INDEX

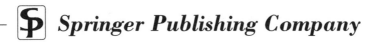

Springer Publishing Company

Structured Group Psychotherapy for Bipolar Disorder
The Life Goals Program

Mark S. Bauer, MD and **Linda McBride,** MSN

Clients who suffer from bipolar disorder will have to cope with significant manic and depressive symptoms throughout their lives. In this volume, Mark Bauer, a psychiatrist, and Linda McBride, a nurse, present a two-phase treatment program designed to improve both illness self-management skills, as well as social and occupational functioning.

> STRUCTURED GROUP PSYCHOTHERAPY FOR BIPOLAR DISORDER
>
> The Life Goals Program
>
> MARK S. BAUER
> LINDA McBRIDE
>
> 𝕊ℙ
>
> SPRINGER PUBLISHING COMPANY

Phase One is a highly structured, five-session psychoeducational program that involves assisting individuals who suffer from bipolar disorder to become more active in learning, thinking, and understanding about their own illness with its unique patterns and problems. Phase Two focuses on helping each group member identify meaningful and realistic life goals that have been interrupted by bipolar disorder. Each client is taught to develop a behavioral plan and to employ cognitive techniques to maximize their chances for success in achieving these life goals. This volume is useful for health care professionals working with clients who suffer from depression and manic depression, including psyhciatrists, psychologists, nurses, and group therapists.

1996   240pp   0-8261-9300-5   hardcover

536 Broadway, New York, NY 10012-3955 • (212) 431-4370 • Fax (212) 941-7842

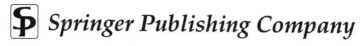
Springer Publishing Company

Case Management in the Treatment of Drug and Alcohol Abuse

Harvey A. Siegal, PhD and **Richard C. Rapp,** MSW

Case managers are in a unique position to coordinate a range of health and social services and offer support to their clients to help them achieve their treatment goals. Based on a special issue of the *Journal of Case Management*, this important book reviews the use and adaptations of case management for the treatment of such special populations as substance abusing women, prisoners, and HIV+ drug users. The chapters provide a well-balanced treatment of the subject including descriptions of innovations in the field, the impact of case management on health care costs, and the challenges faced in the implementation of case management.

Case Management and Substance Abuse Treatment
Practice and Experience

Harvey A. Siegal
Richard C. Rapp
Editors

S SPRINGER PUBLISHING COMPANY

Contents:

- Practical Issues in the Application of Case Management to Substance Abuse Treatment, *M.S. Ridgely*
- Strengths-Based Case Management: A Role in Addressing Denial in Substance Abuse Treatment, *R. C. Rapp, C. W. Kelliher, J. H. Fisher, and F. J. Hall*
- Appropriateness of Assertive Case Management for Drug-Involved Prison Releasees, *J.A. Inciardi, S.S. Martin, and F.R. Scarpitti*
- Case Management Applications in Substance Use Disorders, *M.L. Willenbring*
- Case Management and Community-Based Treatment of Women with Substance Abuse Problems, *W.P. Sullivan*
- Case Management to Enhance HIV Risk Reduction Among Users of Injection Drugs and Crack Cocaine, *R. Falck, R. G. Carlson, S. K. Price, and J. A. Turner*

1995 144pp 0-8261-9170-3 hardcover

536 Broadway, New York, NY 10012-3955 • (212) 431-4370 • Fax (212) 941-7842

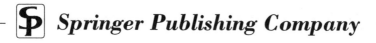
Springer Publishing Company

The Psychological Management of Chronic Pain, Second Edition
A Treatment Manual & Patient's Manual Set

H. Clare Philips, PhD
Stanley Rachman, PhD

Treatment Manual

This newly revised and up-dated volume is a practical guide for clinicians to help their clients manage and alleviate problems associated with chronic pain. Based on the Gate Control Model, the manual gives detailed and structured information to enable the cognitive-behavioral oriented clinician conduct a time-limited,

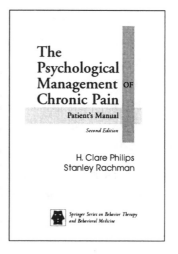

therapist-guided/self-management program. The new edition places an emphasis on the cognitive components of treatment including new chapters on the "new" psychology of pain, memory of pain, the overprediction of pain, pain-related cognitions and how they are measured.

Patient's Manual

Designed to help patients review all the material presented in the course, the Patient's manual contains supplemental information to the nine session course in the main volume. It is invaluable as a resource in difficult times to help patients cope with setbacks.

1995   272pp   0-8261-6113-8   softcover

536 Broadway, New York, NY 10012-3955 • (212) 431-4370 • Fax (212) 941-7842

Springer Publishing Company

The Nurse Consultant's Handbook
Belinda Puetz, PhD, RN
Linda J. Shinn, MBA, RN, CAE

What is a consultant? What type of person makes a successful consultant? How does one launch and manage one's own business as a consultant? This manual answers these questions and provides comprehensive guidelines and practical information on becoming a nurse consultant.

THE NURSE
CONSULTANT'S
HANDBOOK

Belinda Puetz
Linda J. Shinn

SPRINGER PUBLISHING COMPANY

The authors, both experienced consultants, outline the consultation process in detail, describe the business and financial savvy required, and give tips on marketing and pricing one's services, making presentations, networking, and managing one's personal life in relation to one's career. The book addresses independent entrepreneurs as well as "intrapreneurs" who consult as an inside member of a larger organization.

Contents:
- What is Consultation?
- The Consultation Process
- Preparation for Consultation: Planning a Career Path
- The Internal Nurse Consultant
- Starting a Consulting Business
- Marketing Consultation Services
- Networking
- Legal and Ethical Aspects of Consulting
- The Consultant as a Person

1997   248pp   0-8261-9520-2   Hard

536 Broadway, New York, NY 10012-3955 • (212) 431-4370 • Fax (212) 941-7842